T0259081

Palliative Care

Editor

ANGIE MALONE

CRITICAL CARE NURSING CLINICS OF NORTH AMERICA

www.ccnursing.theclinics.com

Consulting Editor
DEBORAH GARBEE

March 2022 • Volume 34 • Number 1

ELSEVIER

1600 John F. Kennedy Boulevard ● Suite 1800 ● Philadelphia, Pennsylvania, 19103-2899

http://www.theclinics.com

CRITICAL CARE NURSING CLINICS OF NORTH AMERICA Volume 34, Number 1
March 2022 ISSN 0899-5885, ISBN-13: 978-0-323-92010-0

Editor: Kerry Holland
Developmental Editor: Ann Gielou M. Posedio

Critical Care Nursing Clinics of North America (ISSN 0899-5885) is published quarterly by Elsevier Inc., 360 Park Avenue South, New York, NY 10010-1710. Months of issue are March, June, September, and December. Business and Editorial Offices: 1600 John F. Kennedy Blvd., Suite 1800, Philadelphia, PA 19103-2899. Periodicals postage paid at New York, NY and additional mailing offices. Subscription prices are $160.00 per year for US individuals, $593.00 per year for US institutions, $100.00 per year for US students and residents, $206.00 per year for Canadian individuals, $611.00 per year for Canadian institutions, $230.00 per year for international individuals, $611.00 per year for international institutions, $115.00 per year for international students/residents and $100.00 per year for Canadian students/residents. To receive student/resident rate, orders must be accompanied by name of affiliated institution, data of term, and the *signature* of program/residency coordinator on institution letterhead. Orders will be billed at individual rate until proof of status is received. Foreign air speed delivery is included in all *Clinics* subscription prices. All prices are subject to change without notice. **POSTMASTER:** Send address changes to *Critical Care Nursing Clinics of North America*, Elsevier Health Sciences Division, Subscription Customer Service, 3251 Riverport Lane, Maryland Heights, MO 63043. **Customer Service: 1-800-654-2452 (US and Canada); 314-447-8871 (outside US and Canada). Fax: 314-447-8029. E-mail:** JournalsCustomerService-usa@elsevier.com **(for print support) and** JournalsOnlineSupport-usa@elsevier.com **(for online support).**

Reprints. For copies of 100 or more of articles in this publication, please contact the Commercial Reprints Department, Elsevier Inc., 360 Park Avenue South, New York, New York, 10010-1710; Tel.: 212-633-3874, Fax: 212-633-3820, and E-mail: reprints@elsevier.com.

Critical Care Nursing Clinics of North America is covered in *MEDLINE/PubMed (Index Medicus), International Nursing Index, Nursing Citation Index, Cumulative Index to Nursing and Allied Health Literature, and RNdex Top 100.*

Contributors

CONSULTING EDITOR

DEBORAH GARBEE PhD, APRN, ACNS-BC, FCNS
Associate Dean for Professional Practice, Community Service and Advanced Nursing Practice, Professor of Clinical Nursing, Louisiana State University Health Sciences Center New Orleans School of Nursing, Louisiana, New Orleans

EDITOR

ANGIE MALONE, DNP, APRN, ACNS-BC, OCN, AOCNS, NE-BC
Director Cancer Services, Cecil B. Highland and Barbara B. Highland Cancer Center, United Hospital Center-WVU Medicine, Bridgeport, West Virginia

AUTHORS

COLETTE D. BAUDOIN, PhD (c), MSN, RN, OCN, CNE
Instructor of Clinical Nursing, School of Nursing, Louisiana State University Health Sciences Center New Orleans, New Orleans, Louisiana

ALEXANDRIA BEAR, MD
Assistant Professor, Department Medicine, Division of Geriatric and Palliative Medicine, Medical College of Wisconsin, Milwaukee, Wisconsin

DAWN M. BLANCHARD, DNP, AGCNS
Fort Huachuca, Arizona

LYNNE BROPHY, MSN, PMGT-BC, APRN-CNS, AOCN
Breast Oncology Clinical Nurse Specialist, The Ohio State University Cancer Comprehensive Center and Richard J. Solove Research Institute, The Ohio State University, Stefanie Spielman Comprehensive Breast Center, Columbus, Ohio

JO CLARKE, DNP, ANP-BC, NP-C, ACNP-BC, APRN-CNP, AOCNP
Inpatient Medical Oncology Nurse Practitioner, Department of Internal Medicine, Division of Medical Oncology, Arthur G. James Hospital and Richard J. Solove Research Institute, The Ohio State University Wexner Medical Center, Columbus, Ohio

KARIN COONEY-NEWTON, MSN, RN, APRN, ACCNS-AG, CCRN
Pulmonary Clinical Nurse Specialist, Bayhealth Medical Center, Dover, Delaware

DELIA M. CORTEZ, MSW, LCSW, LICSW, APHSW-C
Licensed Clinical Social Worker for Palliative Care at UCLA Health, Los Angeles, California

NICOLE E. CROUCH, MSN, RN
Honolulu, Hawaii

JUDY L. CRUZ, MSN, RN
Honolulu, Hawaii

ALISON H. DAVIS, PhD, RN, CNE, CHSE
Associate Professor of Clinical Nursing, School of Nursing, Louisiana State University Health Sciences Center New Orleans, New Orleans, Louisiana
Honolulu, Hawaii

JEANNE M. ERICKSON, PhD, RN
Associate Professor, University of Wisconsin-Milwaukee, College of Nursing, Milwaukee, Wisconsin

RONEL P. ESTORGIO
Honolulu, Hawaii

JILL GUTTORMSON, PhD, RN
Associate Dean for Academic Affairs, Associate Professor, Marquette University, College of Nursing, Milwaukee, Wisconsin

ERIC S. HARDING, MLS
Clinical Services Librarian, Medical College of Wisconsin Libraries, Milwaukee, Wisconsin

ERIN C. HARE, MSN, RN, CCRN
Nursing Professional Development Specialist Medical ICU and Rapid Response Team, ChristianaCare Hospital, Newark, Delaware

CHERYL (MOANA) KAAIALII, MSN, RN
Honolulu, Hawaii

CATHY MAHER-GRIFFITHS, DNS, MSHCM, RN, RNC-OB, NEA-BC
Instructor of Clinical Nursing, Graduate Program, Louisiana State University Health School of Nursing, New Orleans, Louisiana

SEAN MARKS, MD
Associate Professor, Department Medicine, Division of Geriatric and Palliative Medicine, Medical College of Wisconsin, Milwaukee, Wisconsin

NATALIE S. MCANDREW, PhD, RN, ACNS-BC, CCRN-K
Assistant Professor, University of Wisconsin-Milwaukee, College of Nursing, Nurse Scientist, Froedtert & the Medical College of Wisconsin, Froedtert Hospital, Milwaukee, Wisconsin

AIMME JO MCCAULEY, DNP, MSN, RN
Instructor of Clinical Nursing, School of Nursing, Louisiana State University Health Sciences Center New Orleans, New Orleans, Louisiana

JEANNETTE MEYER, MSN, RN, CCRN-K, CCNS, PCCN-K, ACHPN
Clinical Nurse Specialist for Palliative Care at UCLA Health, Los Angeles, California

MERNIE MIYASATO-CRAWFORD, MSSA, LCSW
Honolulu, Hawaii

PATRICIA W. NISHIMOTO, DNS
Honolulu, Hawaii

JOLEEN G. PANGELINAN, BSN, RN
Washington, DC

JAYSHIL PATEL, MD
Associate Professor, Department of Medicine, Division of Pulmonary, Critical Care and Sleep Medicine, Medical College of Wisconsin, Milwaukee, Wisconsin

DOROTHY N. PIERCE, DNP, RN, NP-C, CRN, CBCN, CRNI, CLT
Radiation Oncology, Advanced Practice Nurse, Rutgers Cancer Institute of New Jersey, New Brunswick, New Jersey

DEBORAH RUSSELL, MSN, FNP-BC, APRN-NP, ACHPN
Inpatient Palliative Medicine Nurse Practitioner, Department of Palliative Medicine, Arthur G. James Hospital and Richard J. Solove Research Institute, The Ohio State University Wexner Medical Center, Columbus, Ohio

MICHELE L. WEBER, DNP, RN, APRN-CNS, APRN-NP, CCRN, CCNS, OCN, AOCNS
Oncology Critical Care Clinical Nurse Specialist, Arthur G. James Hospital and Richard J. Solove Research Institute, The Ohio State University Wexner Medical Center, Columbus, Ohio

PHYLLIS WHITEHEAD, PhD, APRN/CNS, ACHPN, PMGT-BC, FNAP, FAAN
Palliative Medicine Clinical Nurse Specialist, Clinical Ethicist, Carilion Roanoke Memorial Hospital Palliative Care Service, Associate Professor, Virginia Tech Carilion School of Medicine, Roanoke, Virginia

LORI JEAN WILLIAMS, DNP, RN, RNC-NIC, CCRN, NNP-BC
Clinical Nurse Specialist, Universal Care Unit and Pediatric Float Team, American Family Children's Hospital, University of Wisconsin Hospitals and Clinics, Madison, Wisconsin

RICHELL, A. VANNIEUWENHUYZEN, BSN, RN
Honolulu, Hawaii

Contents

> The IMPACT-ICU program provides staff with tools that make difficult palliative conversations easier; introduces the "3 conversations," incorporates role-play activities, and provides for continued coaching. This program is highly relevant to the military health system, which typically lacks a specialized palliative care service. It is easily transferable to any environment to include austere locations as well as other disparate health care institutions. Although titled IMPACT-ICU, it uses communication skills that are appropriate for any difficult conversation in any situation, which makes it appropriate for empowering all multidisciplinary team members in any work area.

> Historically, the goal of care in a pediatric or neonatal intensive care unit was to do everything medically possible to cure illness or prolong life. When curative therapies were no longer appropriate, the approach was to turn to end-of-life care. Currently, some children are surviving illnesses that formerly resulted in death or significant disability. Their lives may be viewed as lacking in quality. A palliative care approach can be used in select pediatric populations to improve quality of life, clarify treatment decisions to be aligned with the child's goals and values, and minimize suffering.

> Empirical data show benefits to palliative care (PC) early across the disease trajectory. In the United States, compelling racial inequities exist in access to PC services for minority populations. Minorities who are diagnosed with advanced disease later than nonminorities report adversity accessing treatment availabilities. Thus, poverty, racial discrimination, insurance coverage, and education barriers can affect a person's access to PC assistance. These barriers ultimately result in delayed diagnosis and overall poorer health outcomes. Social and health care inequalities are broad among the sphere of the vulnerable and marginalized minority populations accessing PC.

> Adolescents and young adults (AYAs) may be cared for in a pediatric or adult ICU. Specific needs of AYAs differ from those of populations typically found in either ICU. This review identifies research focused on experiences of AYAs in ICUs, their family members, and the health care professionals who care for them. Limited research about AYAs in ICUs was found (10 articles met inclusion criteria). Findings revealed that AYAs want to be treated as individuals and need health care professionals to partner with them. Further research is needed to inform developmentally appropriate care and improve serious illness communication.

> Homeless individuals are seldom offered the opportunity to complete advance directives and designate decision makers. During a catastrophic illness, health care providers are left to do aggressive, life-prolonging treatments that the patient may not want while seeking decision makers who may not be familiar with the patient or what their wishes would be. The authors spearheaded a program to offer homeless individuals the opportunity to review and complete an advance directive and parlayed that work into a secondary project to provide a comfortable end-of-life experience for homeless patients.

> End of life (EOL) can be an extremely stressful experience for patients, their families, and health care staff. Critical care nurses are trained to help patients survive acute episodes and assist in restoring their health. Unfortunately, not all ICU patients are able to fully recover or obtain previous quality of life before hospitalization. In these situations, the focus moves to transitioning patients from restorative care to palliative care. This article will explain EOL care guidelines for critical care nurses using the Respiratory Distress Observation Scale to ensure patient comfort during compassionate extubation.

> Medicare's new focus on end-of-life care has driven nurses and other clinicians to re-examine when advanced care planning should begin, and serious illness discussions should be conducted. This article will address barriers to, cultural influences on, framing of, and documentation of serious illness discussions using a case study approach.

The COVID-19 pandemic and nursing shortage has impacted new graduate nurse (NGN) careers. Many NGNs gain initial employment with intensive care areas, encountering unprecedented stress due to high patient
acuities, technology, and deaths. Having not yet transitioned into nursing
practice, the NGN can experience a reality shock. Nurses are responsible
for the care of the dying patient in the intensive care setting, despite inconsistencies in undergraduate curricula on death and dying. Nurse residency
programs provide transition-to-practice support and reduce the stressors
experienced by NGNs. Residency programs which specifically include
palliative care and/or end-of-life content can positively impact stress,
burnout, and turnover rates in NGNs.

With the frequency of infant deaths in the United States, many attributed to
congenital malformations and prematurity, the neonatal intensive care unit
(NICU) nurse must be adept at planning and providing perinatal palliative
care. The NICU nurse requires education and training to proficiently
contribute to the care planning and delivery of care and facilitate
memory-making activities. The provision of perinatal palliative care may
precipitate moral distress and needs to be addressed with education
and resilience-fostering activities. To further perinatal palliative care effectiveness, research needs to be conducted.

Dementia is a progressive, incurable condition that causes limitations in
life and should be recognized as a life-limiting condition. Health care professionals should understand its trajectory to better manage symptoms
and to provide early and ongoing advance care planning. Advanced practice registered nurses are uniquely qualified to work with patients and their
families to identify care preferences and then to align treatments to them.
Palliative care and hospice are important interventions that should be integrated into the management of patients with dementia. Additionally, early
integration of palliative medicine can better manage symptoms and lessen
the strain on loved ones.

Palliative Care

CRITICAL CARE NURSING
CLINICS OF NORTH AMERICA

SERIES OF RELATED INTEREST

Nursing Clinics of North America http://www.nursing.theclinics.com

---

THE CLINICS ARE AVAILABLE ONLINE!
Access your subscription at:
www.theclinics.com

Preface

Critical Care Nursing: Expanding the Skill Set in Palliative Care

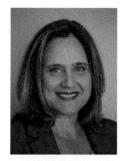

Angie Malone, DNP, APRN, ACNS-BC, OCN, AOCNS, NE-BC
Editor

Health care as we know it has undergone a major change and shift over the last year in part due to the COVID-19 pandemic. As health care providers, we have been forced to reevaluate how we provide care in a more holistic patient-centered manner. Palliative care is even more important to help guide nursing practice to ensure quality care is delivered to patients in all settings, including the intensive care unit (ICU) and other critical care areas. Roughly 20% of people in the United States die in an ICU setting each year and will experience a myriad of debilitating symptoms, such as pain, dyspnea, delirium, or psychological distress.[1] In addition, the ICU consumes 20% of hospital expenditures and is in part due to the aging population and the increasing cost of health care.[2] Palliative care has become increasingly accepted across the health care spectrum as an essential component of comprehensive care in the critical care setting.[3] Now, the focus has shifted somewhat, and critical care nurses must be in tune with concepts that might have otherwise seemed out of place before.

This issue of *Critical Care Nursing Clinics of North America* focuses on providing the critical care nurse with a knowledge base to develop skills to effectively utilize palliative care services and to understand the importance of utilizing palliative care within critical care settings. We begin our issue with the article entitled, "Palliative Care Education for Staff in the Intensive Care Unit/Advanced Practice Registered Nurses (APRNs) and Teamwork in Palliative Care," which describes the importance of providing appropriate education and implementing teamwork among health care teams. In addition, other topics discussed in this issue include minority populations and community/urban populations, the clinical nurse specialist role in palliative care, telehealth, new graduate nurses in the ICU, and end-of-life decisions. It is my intention to provide critical care nurses with expanded knowledge and skills in palliative care to promote a more holistic

Crit Care Nurs Clin N Am 34 (2022) xi–xii
https://doi.org/10.1016/j.cnc.2021.11.011
0899-5885/22/© 2021 Published by Elsevier Inc.

ccnursing.theclinics.com

evidence-based approach to care of patients both while in the critical care setting and along the continuum of care that impacts patient outcomes.

Angie Malone, DNP, APRN, ACNS-BC, OCN, AOCNS, NE-BC
Cecil B. Highland and Barbara B.
Highland Cancer Center
United Hospital Center-WVU Medicine
327 Medical Park Drive
Bridgeport, WV 26330, USA

E-mail address:
maryangiemalone@gmail.com

REFERENCES

1. Gatta B, Turnbull J. Providing palliative care in the medical ICU: a qualitative study of MICU physicians' beliefs and practices. Am J Hosp Palliat Care 2018;35(10): 1309–13.
2. Kyeremanteng K, Gagnon LP, Thavorn K, et al. The impact of palliative care consultation in the ICU on length of stay: a systematic review of cost and evaluation. J Intensive Care Med 2018;33(6):346–53.
3. Mun E, Umbarger L, Ceria-Ulep C, et al. Palliative care processes embedded in the ICU workflow may reserve palliative care teams for refractory cases. Am J Hosp Palliat Care 2018;35(1):60–5.

IMPACT-ICU

A Relevant Sustainable Program for Military Institutions

Dawn M. Blanchard, DNP, AGCNS[a], Joleen G. Pangelinan, BSN, RN[b],
Mernie Miyasato–Crawford, MSSA, LCSW[c],
Patricia W. Nishimoto, DNS[c],*, Nicole E. Crouch, MSN, RN[c],*,
Richell A. Vannieuwenhuyzen, BSN, RN[c],*, Judy L. Cruz, MSN, RN[c],*,
Ronel P. Estorgio[c],*, Cheryl (Moana) Kaaialii, MSN, RN[c],*

KEYWORDS

- Primary palliative care • Communication • Military

KEY POINTS

- IMPACT-ICU is a program that focuses on training primary palliative care through the use of role-playing specific communication tools through the use of the 3 conversations.
- This program is highly relevant to the military health system, which typically lacks a specialized palliative care service. It is easily transferable to any environment to include austere locations as well as other disparate health care institutions.
- Although titled IMPACT-ICU, it uses communication skills that are appropriate for any difficult conversation in any situation, which makes it appropriate for empowering all multi-disciplinary team members in any work area.

INTRODUCTION

Innovative and pragmatic palliative care communication programs are developed each year. But when the author/originator is no longer part of the project, what happens? This question is especially relevant in a military health care environment where staff are moved every 18 to 36 months because of deployments, transfers, and so forth. How is a dynamic program, one that impacts the ability of staff to be able to know and honor patient wishes, sustained? The IMPACT-ICU program (Integrating Multidisciplinary Palliative Care into the ICU) aims to address these difficult challenges. The IMPACT-ICU program provides staff with tools that make difficult

[a] Room O-D-34, Garden Level, 2240 East Winrow Avenue, Fort Huachuca, AZ, USA; [b] 300 5th Avenue, Bldg 62, Washington, DC, USA; [c] 1 Jarrett White Road, Honolulu, HI, USA
* Corresponding authors.
E-mail addresses: patricia.w.nishimoto.civ@mail.mil (P.W.N.); nicole.e.crouch.civ@mail.mil (N.E.C.); richell.a.vannieuwenhuyzen.mil@mail.mil (R.A.V.); judy.l.cruz2.mil@mail.mil (J.L.C.); ronel.p.estorgio.mil@mail.mil (R.P.E.); cheryl.m.kaaialii.civ@mail.mil (C.K.)

Crit Care Nurs Clin N Am 34 (2022) 1–12
https://doi.org/10.1016/j.cnc.2021.11.001
0899-5885/22/© 2022 Elsevier Inc. All rights reserved.

ccnursing.theclinics.com

palliative conversations easier; introduces the "3 conversations," incorporates role-play activities, and provides for continued coaching.

HISTORY/BACKGROUND

Nursing staff at the University of California, San Francisco (UCSF), concerned patients were receiving aggressive life prolonging treatment that they possibly would not have wanted, developed IMPACT-ICU as a strategy for intensive care unit (ICU) nursing staff to learn and explore patient values and beliefs.[1,2] Owing to UCSF's multiple ICUs, there was adequate staff to implement the program.

Dr Virginia Blackman, a Navy nurse, became aware of UCSF's program. Realizing the effect that this program could impart because of a dire need for palliative care and training in military facilities, Dr Blackman received approval of the EBP Implementation Grant from the Tri-Service Nursing Research Program (TSNRP) for development and implementation of the IMPACT-ICU into military treatment facilities. The question remained whether or not this could be accomplished with only 1 to 2 ICUs in military facilities and a smaller number of staff. Her doctoral dissertation focused on that question of efficacy at smaller institutions and the results were resoundingly positive.[3] When she presented her work at the Tri-Service Nursing Research Program (TSNRP) Dissemination Course in 2018, the Army critical care clinical nurse specialist, Major (MAJ) Dawn Blanchard, from Tripler Army Medical Center (TAMC) expressed interest in implementing the program there. In late 2019, Dr Blackman and MAJ Blanchard worked together to coordinate the intricacies of cross-service collaboration to bring Dr Blackman to TAMC.

The TAMC staff were enthusiastic about the idea of bringing the program to Hawaii and quickly undertook the program. The training consisted of 2 separate courses. The first course was designed to specifically train new facilitators. The second course afforded the new facilitators the opportunity to immediately apply what they had learned to mentor new team members under the expert supervision and coaching of Dr Blackman the following day. This was not unusual for the military routine of "see one, do one, teach one" or what is commonly called "hip pocket training."

Several courses were held, with great response from the participants and abundant staff interest. However, during this early stage in the program implementation, the COVID-19 virus began spreading throughout Asia. In response, MAJ Blanchard, instrumental in bringing the program to TAMC and a core facilitator, deployed. This left the rest of the facilitator team responsible for continuing the course, the content of which is described in detail in Blackman and colleagues, 2019.

DISCUSSION
A Need for Primary Palliative Care

In 2015, Military Medicine published an article highlighting the fact that although the military was a "leader in trauma and point of care trauma," they were lacking a robust system addressing palliative care, noting at the time that there were only 2 locations out of 56 Military Health System locations that offered the specialty.[4] The access to specialty palliative care continues to be a concern throughout the MHS system.

TAMC's isolated island location in Hawaii is unlike those on the US mainland and locally (on the economy) available specialty palliative care resources are extremely limited. In addition, when it is available, the military insurance coverage for specialty palliative care by local providers is strictly limited to pediatric patients and those who are veteran affairs beneficiaries (VAB). Currently, military health insurance does not cover civilian specialty supportive care for active duty service members, adult family members, or retirees who may not be VAB. This need for palliative care transcends the boundaries of TAMC as palliative care remains limited throughout the military health system.

Owing to this identified gap in formal specialty palliative care availability at TAMC, there was a recognized need for the palliative care skills to be used by all clinicians, in what is known as primary palliative care. This is consistent with nationwide recognition by the American Nursing Association (ANA), the American Medical Association (AMA), the American Society of Clinical Oncology (ASCO), and the American College of Surgeons (ACS) that all health care providers be able to provide primary palliative care.[5-8] The National Association of Social Workers also published standards for palliative care practice encouraging each clinician to have the skills to provide primary palliative care.[9]

"Recognising when intensive care will not restore a person's health, and helping patients and families embrace goals related to symptom relief, interpersonal connection, or spiritual fulfilment are central challenges of critical care practice."[10] When a patient's condition engenders ambiguity, ambivalence, or conflict with regards to the patient's wishes in the context of the health care team's identified care options, it becomes the nurse's/clinician's role as a patient and family advocate to acknowledge and help navigate that gap through their own primary palliative care skills.

SIGNIFICANCE TO MILITARY NURSING

Most military nurses work without specialized Palliative Care Teams or Services as additional resources.[4] Owing to this fact, the communication skills taught in the IMPACT-ICU course are especially relevant to the military nurse. The skills are portable and easily transferable to any clinical environment, in large or small military Medical Treatment Facilities (MTFs) with varying ranges in ICU bed capacity. Military clinicians are typically assigned to new duty stations as often as every 18 to 36 months and are ascribed or deployed to work in a wide variety of settings, circumstances, and job positions. Oftentimes, military ICU nurses have limited to no experience with serious illness, suffering, and dying leaving them inadequately prepared to meet the needs of those patients and their families through advocacy. This is also the case with the medical-surgical nurses, who often have even less clinical experience than their ICU counterparts. Deployed military staff often work in austere environments lacking the clinical infrastructures or resources found in MTFs. IMPACT-ICU skills do not require any particular external organizational, institutional, or financial specifications to be applied effectively. The only requirement is a personal commitment on the part of each participant and facilitator to learn and apply the new skills with confidence.

The IMPACT-ICU course targets its approach by empowering the individual nurse and other members of the health care team to focus on patient wishes and values as equal and valued team members. It has been shown to benefit the military because it helps the individual develop in both a personal and professional way that can flourish positive improvement in leadership skills. Thus, IMPACT-ICU's focus on personal empowerment and teamwork supports the larger military goal of readiness as a soldier, sailor, or airman. Clinicians both stateside and "down-range" in a deployed environment can have high-quality and purposeful conversations that foster relations between interdisciplinary team members and the patient's loved ones.

EXPANDING THE VISION TO MEET THE NEEDS

Evidence shows that learning and applying IMPACT-ICU communication skills enhance the effectiveness of each individual practitioner of primary palliative care.[5–17] When adapting IMPACT-ICU to military health care, Dr Blackman modified the 3 discussion scenarios to be military-focused, yet still ICU-focused. Immediate recognition by the TAMC faculty of the value of this program and the need for upstreaming primary palliative care discussions created the opportunity to open this to non-ICU nurses, that is, those working on the general medical/surgical wards, in clinics, and even the emergency department setting. The prospect of expansion also included ancillary professional staff and nonprofessional staff. Although originally designed specifically for the ICU nurses, the conversations in IMPACT-ICU exemplified critical communication skills to optimize patient care in any setting, by any clinician; the vision for expansion was born and embraced as worthy by all. The expansion at first branched out to the medical-surgical areas, then encompassed the emergency department. Although expanded in scope, these workshops initially remained true to the "3 conversations" that focused on an adult in the ICU. Workshop comments and surveys results indicated that participants enthusiastically embraced the course. Each workshop offered expanded the vision a little farther and facilitators found that including participants from other expanded clinical areas and disciplines (social workers, physicians, chaplains, respiratory therapists, medical support assistants, medics, nursing assistants, psychologists, and dieticians) reaped even *more* benefits to the participants and program.

Eventually, a pediatric nurse and an oncology pediatric resident attended and asked that a workshop with specific pediatric role-plays be designed. Prognosis-related questions are often asked of pediatric nurses and developing skills as part of a team are essential for providing consistent support to families.[18] MAJ Blanchard contacted UCSF to ask if a pediatric-specific course had been created and when learning it had not, received permission to again modify the 3 conversation scenarios to meet that gap. Several pediatric clinicians worked diligently to develop a scenario fitting the "3 conversations" format, using a pertinent pediatric content and design. The ensuing pediatric-based course was conducted with participants that included nursing aides, respiratory therapists, child life specialists, nurses, and physicians working on the pediatric ward and the Pediatric Intensive Care Unit. The feedback found that the course was relevant and seen as immediately applicable (**Figs. 1–3**).

Shortly after implementation of this program, a new coronavirus, SARS-CoV-2, known as COVID-19, was identified and began taking hold in Asia. As it continued to spread throughout the world, the need for the IMPACT-ICU became even more imperative to the facilitators left at TAMC who were passionate about sharing these relevant tools with all team members. The pandemic on the horizon highlighted the need that all clinicians to be prepared to maximize their communication skills surrounding inescapable difficult conversations.[11]

Two key initial IMPACT-ICU facilitators, an experienced social worker and a seasoned oncology palliative care Clinical Nurse Specialist, who had participated in countless palliative care family conference meetings, rapidly stepped up and became key to the proliferation and sustainment of the program. Owing to their influence and guidance, the team began to earnestly recruit interdisciplinary team members to include social workers, physicians, and chaplains and to promulgate the program throughout the health care facility. One of many postworkshop comments reinforced the value of this interdisciplinary team, *"Working with the interdisciplinary team opened my eyes to advocate for my patient."*

From its conception, social workers have valued interdisciplinary teamwork as integral to the patient's success. Having a social worker as a key facilitator proved to be influential to the sustainment of IMPACT-ICU at TAMC. She helped solidify the team because of her professional training and ability to build relationships, navigate

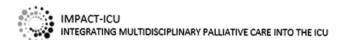

IMPACT-ICU
INTEGRATING MULTIDISCIPLINARY PALLIATIVE CARE INTO THE ICU

Pediatric Role Play Case Handout

ROLE PLAY #1: ELICITING FAMILY PERSPECTIVES AND NEEDS
NURSE (LEAD) ROLE

Janet Smith is a 6 year-old female who was admitted to the PICU yesterday from the ED. She presented with uncoordinated movements, headaches, vision disturbances, and had two episodes of emesis. She has a past medical history of being an ex 30 week premature infant. Lab work was unremarkable, but a head CT and MRI displayed a brain mass located on the brainstem. She showed evidence of respiratory compromise with intermittent slowed breathing and apneic periods and was started on a non-invasive ventilation system upon admission to the PICU.

You are the bedside nurse caring for Janet for the first time this morning. Overnight, her apneic episodes became more frequent despite non-invasive ventilation and she was emergently intubated.

You hear that Janet's mother has been at her bedside since admission. You learn that she is a single parent without any extended family, and derives her support from friends. You and the night nurse agree about the importance of beginning to address prognosis and goals of care. After report, you enter the patient's room and introduce yourself to Janet's mother, Ms. Sarah Smith.

- -

ROLE PLAY #1: ELICITING FAMILY PERSPECTIVES AND NEEDS
FAMILY (SUPPORTING) ROLE

You are Sarah Smith, a 40 year old single mother to Janet Smith. You don't have any extended family and receive support through friends. Janet is your daughter who was diagnosed with a brain tumor. She was an ex 30 week premature infant that spent two month in the Neonatal ICU. She had been doing fairly well until yesterday where she had was more clumsy that usual, she was complaining that her head hurts and that everything seemed blurry, and you took her to the Emergency Department for evaluation where she also vomited twice. She was admitted to the Pediatric ICU where she had periods that she wasn't breathing and was eventually placed on a breathing machine overnight. You have been at your child's bedside since admission and are feeling exhausted and overwhelmed.

It is now morning, and you woke up from a short nap. The day shift nurse enters your child's room and introduces herself|

Your understanding of your child's prognosis is: You have been given an extensive update from her nurses and doctors. You understand that she has a tumor on her brainstem that it is affecting Janet's ability to breathe on her own. You find this information concerning, but don't understand what it all means. You are hoping she will receive treatment that will help remove or "cure" the tumor or help her recover so that she can go home.

If asked what she is like as a person and how you feel about certain treatments: She is a "miracle baby" and a "survivor" and "so full of life". You believe in modern medicine and its ability to save just about anyone. Janet has already been an example of a "miracle" and you believe that she can do it again. You feel that you have to try every option otherwise you will always wonder if you could have done more or feel as if you "gave up on your child".

Fig. 1. Eliciting family perspectives and needs.

systems, and by representing social workers' skills to holistically assess and understand individuals within their larger contexts of life. The addition of the social worker role allowed for the team to embrace and learn from their professional skills; therapeutic counseling, advocacy, and conflict resolution as well as through the sharing of their unique professional experiences, outlook, perspectives, and expectations.

The clinical roles of the facilitators added depth and meaning to the IMPACT-ICU learners' experience, the communication skills taught, demonstrated and practiced

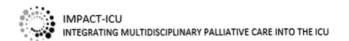

IMPACT-ICU
INTEGRATING MULTIDISCIPLINARY PALLIATIVE CARE INTO THE ICU

ROLE PLAY #2: WORKING WITH PHYSICIANS TO ADDRESS FAMILY NEEDS
NURSE (LEAD) ROLE

After introducing yourself and completing your morning assessment, you engage in conversation with Ms. Smith, Janet's mother. You learned that she is very concerned about her daughter's condition, but doesn't have a sense of what to expect moving forward. She would like "honest information from the doctor" about her child's status and what treatment options are available. Regarding mom's goals of care, she is adamant that her child is a "survivor" and that she can "beat this thing".

You are worried about the grave prognosis that Janet is likely to have, and how it will affects mom's hopes and beliefs for treatment and recovery. You feel it is important that Ms. Smith receive realistic information about the risk of death or permanent functional impairment. While you feel that continuing the current level of care is appropriate given the fairly new diagnosis, you want to make sure that Ms. Smith, you, and the physician begin to discuss Janet's prognosis and goals of care.

After your discussion with Ms. Smith, she decides to go get a cup of coffee and breakfast. You begin charting when you see Dr. Jones coming to check on your patient. Before he enters the room, he asks you "How are things going?"

- -

ROLE PLAY #2: WORKING WITH PHYSICIANS TO ADDRESS FAMILY NEEDS
PHYSICIAN (SUPPORTING) ROLE

You are Dr. Jones, Janet's attending physician, and have been caring for her since her admission to the PICU yesterday. You have been concerned about the severity of illness and prognosis. With the placement of the tumor on the brainstem, the treatment options are limited and she has a high risk of in-hospital mortality. If she does survive this admission, she will have a prolonged recovery, will never return to her previous functional status, and will eventually experience death in the very near future.

Prior to intubating Janet, your team verified that Ms. Smith, Janet's mother, desired all available treatment for her child. Though there has been no formal family meeting, you have spoken with Ms. Smith several times since admission providing updates on her child's status. You feel you have been very clear and thorough about the severity of her illness and respiratory failure.

In the morning, you decide to check in on the patient. When you arrive at the room, you first check in with his nurse, "How are things going?"

Fig. 2. Working with physicians to address family needs.

as part of IMPACT-ICU symbiotically reinforce and add more instruments to the clinician's toolkit. IMPACT-ICU skills further strengthen their ability to achieve effective engagement, trust-building, interviewing, assessment, and therapeutic alliances with patients and their families—even more essential in the face of the stressors impacting practice. In fact, as far back as 2004, the National Association of Social Workers (NASW) published "Professional Standards for Palliative Care and End of Life Practice," which included Interdisciplinary Teamwork as one of its practice standards, stating "they have the opportunity to influence a range of professionals, consumers, and laypersons regarding life-limiting illness, care of the dying, and the bereaved."[19] Social work's inclusion and involvement in IMPACT-ICU training is a natural evolutionary step.

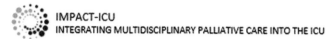
IMPACT-ICU
INTEGRATING MULTIDISCIPLINARY PALLIATIVE CARE INTO THE ICU

ROLE PLAY #3: THE FAMILY MEETING
NURSE (LEAD) ROLE

Dr. Taylor told you that he was very worried about Janet's placement of her brain tumor. He would not be surprised if Janet passed away during this hospitalization. If Janet does recover sufficiently to be discharged from the hospital, she is likely to have permanent functional impairment and will eventually succumb to death in the very near future.

Dr. Taylor agreed to attend a family meeting with you to discuss this information with Ms. Smith. When Ms. Smith comes back to the bedside after her coffee and breakfast, you tell her that you would like to sit down with her and Dr. Taylor to talk about how her child is doing. She said she would be grateful.

You arranged to meet together in a conference room near the PICU.

- -

ROLE PLAY #3: THE FAMILY MEETING
PHYSICIAN (SUPPORTING) ROLE

After talking with Janet's nurse, you agreed to meet with her and Ms. Smith to give an update on her child's condition. You are happy to do this, though you feel you've already relayed the severity of Janet's illness to Ms. Smith.

You will take the initial lead in this meeting, asking Ms. Smith what she understands and then giving her information about her child's condition. When you give information to Ms. Smith, you use medical terms such as "respiratory failure", "grave prognosis", and "high risk of in-hospital mortality."

You will also ask Ms. Smith about whether she would want to continue on the ventilator, though you will not inquire about her idea of quality of life or goals of care.

- -

ROLE PLAY #3: THE FAMILY MEETING
FAMILY (SUPPORTING) ROLE

When you talked with Janet's nurse, she asked you to attend a meeting to talk with her and Dr. Taylor, your child's attending physician, for an update.

Your understanding of your child's prognosis is: You are concerned that she is on the breathing machine. You have been given updates from Dr. Taylor, who was clear that your child is very sick. She looks very sick to you, but you are hoping the tumor can be treated and that Janet will recover to her previous status.

- In the meeting, if you are given information about your child's status using only medical terms, you will not understand it. However, you won't state that you don't understand unless asked.

If asked how you feel about certain treatments: You believe in modern medicine and its ability to save just about anyone.

If asked what your child is like as a person: She is a "fighter" and can "beat this thing." She is your "miracle baby" who is rambunctious, smart, and so full of life. She loves reading stories together and playing outside.

Your emotions: You express worry about your child. If told that she might die or will have permanent functional disability, you become upset. If asked about taking her off the ventilator, you become overwhelmed.

Fig. 3. The family meeting.

A physician learner turned facilitator who was recruited from the first interdisciplinary workshop embraced the value of expanding the program from primarily nursing staff to an interdisciplinary course. Interactive sharing across disciplines and settings resulted in the realization and acknowledgment of commonly experienced anxieties, perceptions, and approaches, as well as greater understanding about the unique challenges each discipline and/or setting brings to the table. Physician participants gained the insight that prognoses given to patients and families often result in the nurses reinforcing and supporting the families as they begin to cope with that information.[15] In other words, the experience of training in an interdisciplinary fashion *in and of itself* generated insights to inform future and ongoing collaborative teamwork.

Chaplain participation helped link the physical, mental, and spiritual health components of palliative care.[20] Plato stated, "...neither ought you to attempt to cure the body without the soul".[21] More often than not, a serious illness and prognosis can cause patients to ask spiritual questions and think profoundly about one's humanity: *who am I and why am I here on earth?* These questions surface not only in patients but also in family members as they contemplate the suffering of a loved one. Chaplains with their distinctive training are invaluable partners in exploring conversations about the meaning of life, suffering, forgiveness, dying, legacy, and so forth.

As part of the IMPACT-ICU interdisciplinary team, the Chaplain helps learners to recognize and respond to spiritual needs. When caregivers understand that the key to responding is not theological solutions, rather authenticity and vulnerability, then it helps them feel more at ease to engage in spiritual conversations when they arise. One postworkshop comment stated *"The Chaplain's involvement made a difference especially with patients who ask if they're going to go to heaven."* Discussions of hope can be realistic when team members are truthful and kindhearted, which can greatly contribute to a patient's quality of life. There can still be healing even if there is no cure. Spiritual support can alleviate emotional distress and soothe the soul and spirit of patients and their families.

However, it is not only the patients and families that need spiritual care, but staff members as well. A component of the IMPACT-ICU Course focuses on self-care. The faculty realized that many of the participants, when asked about their strategies for self-care, listed spirituality. The Chaplain facilitator helped build on this dimension of self-care.

The diversity in clinical roles of the faculty added depth and meaning to IMPACT-ICU learners' experience. The communication skills and perspectives taught, demonstrated, and practiced by each individual faculty member symbiotically reinforced those of the others, and served to add more instruments to each learner's toolkit.

OUTCOMES

TAMC's experience has proven the maxim: "The whole is greater than the sum of its parts" by expanding the impact of an already proven effective resource across different disciplines. The skills and the training are clear, accessible, and easily incorporated by each individual discipline in its own distinctive way. The communication skills and its message of individual empowerment speak to each member of the team in powerfully positive ways. As a cohort, those trained in this manner acquire a "Shared Mental Model"—*across disciplines*—of the importance of primary palliative care practice. Built-in barriers that often exist between disciplines with different perspectives and approaches are greatly diminished because of the common language learned and the mutuality of intent that are engendered during the training experience.

A valuable impact of the course was the focus on the value of communication in improving patient care. In the busy clinical setting, "value" is often assessed by the amount of physical workload produced. It can be very task-oriented. Listening is often not seen as real work. Participants have learned to embrace that the same letters that spell "listen" also are the same letters as "silent." They now make the time to stop, listen, and support patients questioning their goals of care. The postworkshop comments reinforced how this workshop raised the confidence of the participants to engage in palliative conversations (**Box 1**).

Box 1
Postworkshop Comments

"I was not comfortable talking about palliative care but now I have confidence to speak and advocate for my patient and their family members.

"I don't feel confident initiating a meeting between the MD, family, and nurse. But NOW I understand the need for working on behalf of the patient and the family members."

"Being in safe setting where no one judged you made it easier for me to practice the skills and role play."

"The different perspectives of communication between the nurse, patient, and the physicians was an eye-opener"

I *can initiate the process and we are one whole team to accomplish patient goals. I am truly an advocate for the patient*

" I definitely learned the value of family meetings and how important communication skills are".

Understanding different roles of other team members such as the chaplain, sw, pt, rt.

IMPACT ICU brought the process full circle and reinforced understanding of the vital role we all play in palliative care for all of our patients.

"As a physician, it helped me to see the problems from another perspective, and take a second to be present."

Participant turned facilitator. *"I didn't have a definition of palliative care and thought it was something that occurred during terminal disease only." - SW*

IMPACT-ICU is designed to use a pre-evaluation and postevaluation assessment of participants. During this implementation period, 71 learners assessed their confidence in their abilities to use the "3 conversations"; eliciting the family perspectives and needs, working with physicians to address family needs, and active participation in the family meeting. When comparing the 5 different evaluation questions, all workshop participants reported significant improvement in confidence (**Table 1**).

Before IMPACT-ICUs implementation at TAMC, the palliative care nurse's consults primarily originated from the physicians and late in the patients' hospital stay. The inpatient caseload mix was 30% palliative care but now since the implementation of IMPACT-ICU course, the caseload mix is 70% palliative care. Consults now are being placed early in the patients' stay and from a variety of interdisciplinary team members. One facilitator related "I have noticed a behavioral change in the team members that we have mentored. Instead of young nurses asking me (the palliative care nurse) to intervene when a patient expresses their desire to forego aggressive treatment, I now am frequently stopped in order for them to articulate how they used IMPACT-ICU skills and were able to speak with the physician to advocate for the patient" (Patricia W. Nishimoto, DNS, FAAN, email communication, July 14, 2021).

IMPACT-ICU is a highly adaptable and sustainable program. The program consists of a 1-day training workshop that requires minimal preparation and contains valuable communication techniques that can be used not only with patients but also in everyday conversations. In-services can be provided to staff at least annually to help refresh skills. The training day begins with an introduction of why the program was developed and the need for the skill set, followed by a brief discussion defining palliative care. Most of the day consists of role-playing three critical conversations that allow participants to practice the communication skills between nurse-family

Table 1
Preworkshop and postworkshop evaluations

Evaluation Question		Preworkshop				Postworkshop			
1. Assess a family's understanding of a patient's prognosis and goals of care	Scale:	1	2	3	4	1	2	3	4
	# of participants	12	21	35	3	0	4	50	17
2. Arrange a meeting between a patient's family and clinicians to discuss prognosis and goals of care	Scale:	1	2	3	4	1	2	3	4
	# of participants	8	18	38	7	0	2	48	21
3. Contribute to discussions of prognosis and goals of care during family meetings	Scale:	1	2	3	4	1	2	3	4
	# of participants	8	23	31	9	0	4	43	24
4. Arrange a consultation from the palliative care team	Scale:	1	2	3	4	1	2	3	4
	# of participants	19	20	20	12	0	4	44	23
5. Cope with the stresses of working in the ICU or with dying patients	Scale:	1	2	3	4	1	2	3	4
	# of participants	12	22	28	9	0	10	38	23

Number of participants = 71.
Participation measurement:
Scale: 1 to 4.
1 = not confident, 2 = somewhat confident, 3 = confident, and 4 = very confident.

member, nurse-doctor, and during a family meeting in a safe, positive learning environment. The training day ends with a section focused on spiritual care and self-care.

At TAMC, the training of new faculty initially proved difficult. Faculty turnover is high because of the dynamics of military service, and required adaptations. New faculty are now recruited from among class participants, based on the nature and level of engagement and interest exhibited during training. Each recruit is then provided on-the-job education and coaching in subsequent classes and during faculty meetings. Although turnover was initially seen as a challenge, it has proven to be an advantage to the program's sustainment across other MTFs. TAMC's faculty roster includes those who were participants and/or faculty in other MTFs. Thus, IMPACT-ICU continues to grow and spread. The quality of the IMPACT-ICU course has been maintained through the incorporation of other disciplines and through the transition of staff. Expanding the program to other disciplines has created a cohesive team with a shared mental model, which will continue to develop and strengthen all MTFs throughout the military health system.

In addition to teaching participants to improve on naturally engaging and therapeutic communication techniques, with tools that are easily implemented into everyday conversations, IMPACT-ICU also teaches and emphasizes interdisciplinary teamwork. Increasingly, health care organizations face constant pressures to save or cut costs, often evidenced in targets to reduce lengths of stay, reduce staffing levels, and/or shrink services or programs. At the same time, administrative demands are felt to be increasing. Meanwhile, overlapping or unclear role definitions and increased workload stressors at every level often operate to constrain interdisciplinary collaboration. In this environment of care, the need for effective teamwork can be seen as even more essential. These challenges act to highlight IMPACT-ICU's relevance—at the individual level, in its reinforcement of the clinician's desire to provide "patient care," not "paper care," but also at the organizational level, in its enhancement of interdisciplinary teamwork and collaboration.

CLINICS CARE POINTS

- Communication leads to better outcomes for all involved
- Optimal patient advocacy results from communication skills that empower nurses to have the important conversations
- IMPACT-ICU is not just for the ICU—anyone wanting to improve on communication skills will benefit
- IMPACT-ICU is a portable, easily sustainable, and a low investment program with a high return

DISCLOSURE

The authors have nothing to disclose.

REFERENCE

1. Anderson WG, Puntillo K, Boyle D, et al. ICU bedside nurses' involvement in palliative care communication: a multicenter survey. J Pain Symptom Manage 2016; 51(3):589–96.e2.
2. Anderson WG, Puntillo K, Cimino J, et al. Palliative care professional development for critical care nurses: a multicenter program. Am J Crit Care 2017; 26(5):361–71.

3. Blackman V, Hipszer S, Milic M, et al. Recruiting the military to IMPACT-ICU palliative care. Crit Care Med 2019;47(1):393.
4. Snyder S. Palliative care in the U.S. military health system. Mil Med 2015;180(10): 1024–6.
5. American nurses association and hospice & palliative nurses association call for palliative care in every setting. American nurses Association website. 2017. Available at: https://www.nursingworld.org/news/news-releases/2017-news-releases/ american-nurses-association-and-hospice–palliative-nurses-association-call-for-palliative-care-in-every-setting/. Accessed July 1, 2021.
6. Ray A, Najmi A, Sadasivam B. Integrating palliative care with primary care: a synergistic mix. J Fam Med Prim Care 2019;8(9):3074–5.
7. McCormick E, Chai E, Meier DE. Integrating palliative care into primary care. Mt Sinai J Med 2012;79(5):579–85. https://doi.org/10.1002/msj.21338.
8. Sigman M. American College of Surgeons. Practicing primary palliative care: a call to action. FACS.org. 2019. Available at: https://bulletin.facs.org/2019/11/ practicing-primary-palliative-care-a-call-to-action/. Accessed July 5, 2021.
9. NASW standards for palliative & end of life care. National Association of social workers (NASW) Org. 2017. Available at: https://www.naswpress.org/product/ 53608/nasw-standards-for-palliative-amp-end-of-life-care. Accessed July 10, 2021.
10. Turnbull AE, Bosslet GT, Kross EK. Aligning use of intensive care with patient values in the USA: past, present, and future. Lancet Respir Med 2019;7(7): 626–38.
11. Bowman BA, Back AL, Esch AE, et al. Crisis symptom management and patient communication protocols are important tools for all clinicians responding to COVID-19. J Pain Symptom Manage 2020;60(2):e98–100.
12. Boyle DA, Barbour S, Anderson W, et al. Palliative care communication in the ICU: Implications for an oncology-critical care nursing partnership. Semin Oncol Nurs 2017;33(5):544–54.
13. Delgado SA. Increasing nurses' palliative care communication skills. Am J Crit Care 2017;26(5):372.
14. Ferrell B, Buller H, Paice JA. Communication skills: use of the interprofessional communication curriculum to address physical aspects of care. Clin J Oncol Nurs 2020;24(5):547–53.
15. Milic MM, Puntillo K, Turner K, et al. Communicating with patients' families and physicians about prognosis and goals of care. Am J Crit Care 2015;24(4):e56–64.
16. Watson A, Weaver M, Jacobs S, et al. Interdisciplinary communication: documentation of advance care planning and end-of-life care in adolescents and young adults with cancer. J Hosp Palliat Nurs 2019;21(3):215–22.
17. Boyle DA, Anderson WG. Enhancing the communication skills of critical care nurses: focus on prognosis and goals of care discussions. J Clin Outcomes Manag 2015;22(12):543–9.
18. Newman AR, Haglund K, Rodgers CC. Pediatric oncology nurses' perceptions of prognosis-related communication. Nurs Outlook 2019;67(1):101–14.
19. NASW standard for palliative & end of life care . National Association of social workers (NASW) Org. 2000. Available at: https://www.socialworkers.org/ LinkClick.aspx?fileticket=xBMd58VwEhk%3D&portalid=0. Accessed July 7, 2021.
20. Gijsberts MHE, Liefbroer AI, Otten R, et al. Spiritual care in palliative care: a systematic review of the recent European literature. Med Sci (Basel) 2019;7(2):25.
21. Plato. Charmides. In: dialogues of plato: with analyses and introductions1. Charles Scribner's Sons; 2012. p. 3–33.

Palliative Care and Population Management

Utilization of Palliative Care in Pediatric Critical Care Nursing

Lori Jean Williams, DNP, RN, RNC-NIC, CCRN, NNP-BC*

KEYWORDS

- Pediatric palliative care • Pediatric end-of-life care • Family-centered care

KEY POINTS

- Of the estimated 6.3 million children who die each year needing palliative care, reportedly 10% receive it.
- As we understand the complexity of the lived experience of life with chronic medical conditions we have come to appreciate the need for clarity regarding goals of care over time.
- Working with the child and family to set care goals helps to empower the patient, family and care team to maintain the dual goals of cure and comfort.
- Medical therapies that no longer provide benefit may need to be modified or discontinued.
- Desired interventions should be clarified with each encounter so care remains consistent with the child/family's values and goals.

BACKGROUND

In recent years, the complexity of hospitalized pediatric patients has increased. This has been demonstrated by the Healthcare Cost & Utilization Project, which analyzed national trends in the hospitalization rates of children with chronic conditions from 1991 to 2005.[1] Study results showed that the hospitalization rates for children with more than one complex chronic condition increased from 83.7 per 100,000 to 166 per 100,000 admissions ($P<.001$). A recent study of palliative care allocation among intensive care (non–newborn intensive care unit) pediatric admissions in American children's hospitals from 2007 to 2018 reported 1% to 36% of admissions had a palliative care consult.[2] Consultation was found to be low, with considerable variation and inequity across the 52 children's hospitals studied. Utilization was reported to be

Universal Care Unit & Pediatric Float Team, American Family Children's Hospital, University of Wisconsin Hospitals and Clinics, Madison, WI, USA
* American Family Children's Hospital 1675 Highland Avenue Room 7404, Mail Code 0700 Madison, WI 53792.
E-mail address: Lwilliams3@uwhealth.org

Crit Care Nurs Clin N Am 34 (2022) 13–18
https://doi.org/10.1016/j.cnc.2021.11.009

increasing and was independently associated with older age of the child, female sex, having government insurance, having in-hospital mortality, and intensive care–specific palliative care or complex chronic conditions.[2] Of the estimated 6.3 million children who die each year needing palliative care, reportedly 10% receive it because palliative care is not available where the child lives.[3]

PEDIATRIC PALLIATIVE CARE

When the words palliative care are used, parents and health care workers typically think about the transition in care from curative interventions to interventions that address end-of-life issues when cure is no longer possible or probable. The physical and emotional comfort of the child and family is prioritized over efforts to prolong life. Historically, the transition may come very late if at all in the course of a child's illness. I am pleased to share that in the past 20 years of my professional career, there has been a change. As we understand the complexity of the lived experience of children and families with chronic medical conditions, we have come to appreciate the need for communication and clarity regarding goals of care over time.[4] The introduction of "family-centered care" in the early 2000s brought recommendations to build partnerships between parents and the health care team. Domains of family-centered care include:[5,6]

1. Support of the family as a unit
2. Communication with the child and family regarding treatment plans and goals
3. Shared decision-making
4. Incorporation of family values, needs, and preferences into care
5. Relief of symptoms
6. Continuity of care
7. Grief and bereavement support

These domains overlap with priorities that parents identified in a qualitative study of recommendations for end-of-life care.[7] Parents whose children died after withdrawal of support identified 6 priorities—honest and complete information, ready access to staff, communication, care coordination, emotional expression and support by staff, faith, and preservation of the integrity of the parent-child relationship.[7] Over time, palliative care has changed to care based on need, not prognosis.[8] Goals have changed to improve communication, provide support for patients and families, and alleviate physical and emotional symptoms regardless of disease stage.[8–10] Palliative care has become much broader than end-of-life care. Pediatric hospital-based palliative care teams now deal with very diverse medical conditions and longer survival durations than teams caring for adult patients.[11]

Although palliative care principles are the same across patient populations, implementation of pediatric palliative care is different for several reasons. These reasons include the varied emotional maturity and cognitive abilities of the patient, differences in emotional and psychological patient concerns, differences in the etiology of the life-threatening illness, the necessity of including the child and possibly siblings along with parents when making decisions, and the reality that parents not the patient make care decisions.[12]

Palliative care is ideal to integrate into the care of any child with a life-threatening or limiting condition. These conditions include cancer, some congenital heart diseases, and end-organ failure where cure may be possible, but also may fail. Other conditions such as cystic fibrosis, progressive neuromuscular diseases, and severe immunodeficiencies offer long-term treatment to maintain some quality of life for conditions that are chronic and potentially progressive. A newer population of children receiving palliative care are children with nonprogressive and irreversible conditions (such as cerebral palsy, hypoxic brain injury, congenital brain malformations, severe developmental disability, genetic or congenital disease) who are vulnerable to complications of their conditions over time. A changing perspective is the use of palliative care for children who have progressive conditions such as trisomy 13 or 18, or osteogenesis imperfecta type II without a cure currently. As the disease trajectory changes with the advent of new therapies, management may shift from palliative care to cure. There are many examples of novel therapies that are changing the way we look at diseases where there used to be no hope for families. Gene therapies currently available for spinal muscular atrophy type 1, for example, have changed how we discuss prognosis for this disease.[13] Palliative care and ongoing support aid decision-making because these novel therapies are so new, many are experimental, and outcomes are variable.[12]

Many children and families are offered palliative care when all other therapies have been exhausted and there is no hope of a cure. Ideally, palliative care would be offered at the time of diagnosis so that quality of life, relief of symptoms, and optimized days of life can be the focus of management.[12] The timing of diagnosis may occur before the child is born. Prenatal palliative care can assist parents who are forced to make decisions when a life-threatening diagnosis is presented or a disease-modifying treatment for a chronic condition no longer provides benefit.[12]

Palliative care should be considered and perhaps part of the recommended consults when a child with a chronic condition is admitted to the hospital. This care becomes important when symptom management becomes difficult, when difficult decisions need to be made, and when declines in health status over time become evident necessitating discussions to clarify goals of care. Introducing palliative care at this point may give parents the perception that the health care team has given up hope, has nothing more to offer, and believe that current interventions are no longer appropriate or may be causing suffering. The palliative care team can be instrumental in helping children and families understand illness/injury and its potential outcome. They are also well equipped to help explore hopes for a good outcome along with fears of a bad one. Working with the child and family to set care goals helps to empower the patient, family, and care team to maintain the dual goals of cure and comfort. Although advanced care planning is better suited for a time when the patient is well, and includes the patient's primary care provider, anticipatory guidance can be provided if the family needs help to think about their goals of care and begin to develop a care plan as the disease progresses. Care providers may be reluctant to initiate difficult conversations about adding palliative care as an intervention, but research has shown that the integration of palliative care does not lessen a parent's sense of hope.[14] Clinical information that the care team may consider upsetting is the information regarding parents' desire and need to make effective decisions regarding their child's care.[15] Parents who are unable to describe the quality of life for their child tend to choose intense and invasive interventions that may cause suffering near the end of life.[16,17]

INCLUDING THE CHILD IN DECISION-MAKING

Parents are the legal decision makers regarding the treatment of their children, including the introduction of palliative or hospice care services. However, children should be involved in the discussion as developmentally and cognitively appropriate. Young children can voice their preferences and are able to better understand what is happening to them when they are appropriately prepared to engage in discussion. Understanding also facilitates their comfort and reduces anxiety. It is important to explore what relationships and activities are important to the child and how often these continue to be enjoyed as disease or disability progresses. It is also important to understand what the child perceives as suffering. Medical therapies that no longer provide a benefit may need to be modified or discontinued. Life-sustaining measures such as intubation, ventilation, chest compressions, and defibrillation can always be provided when needed, but these interventions may not be compatible with a child's values or goal of care. They also may not result in a desired outcome. Thoughts about these interventions can and do change over time as children become more aware of their disease course and the impact of intervention on their life. Desired interventions should be clarified with each inpatient admission, so care remains consistent with the child/family's values and goals. Children over the age of 18 years may require a health care proxy to make decisions if they are unable to make or communicate decisions. Parents can be assisted in identifying a proxy and completing the necessary documentation, so the child's goals of care and preferences are continued if/when parents are not involved.

SYMPTOM MANAGEMENT

An overlooked benefit of palliative care is their expertise in symptom management, including pain, dyspnea, fatigue, nausea/vomiting, anorexia/weight loss, anxiety, agitation, depression, seizures, secretion management, and sleep disturbance.[18–20] Use of templated orders or algorithms can assist management when symptoms escalate. They also reduce inconsistencies in care as providers change, or providers who may be unfamiliar try to manage symptoms in the palliative care context.

Nonpharmacological interventions such as massage, heat, cold, physical and occupational therapy, meditation, distraction, and guided imagery are an essential part of symptom management.[12] Complementary and alternative therapies such as aromatherapy, healing touch, and hypnosis are also being used and found to be efficacious to improve symptom management.

ADDITIONAL BENEFITS OF PALLIATIVE CARE CONSULTATION

A well-rounded palliative care team can be instrumental in keeping goals of care up-to-date with each admission. This can be accomplished with a check-in upon admission and throughout the hospital course to ensure goals are consistent with the child/family's values or modified as needed. Consistent goals may assist perceptions of satisfaction during the hospitalization. The team can be a valuable source of support to acknowledge stress and split priorities as parents try to balance work, home life, and other children with the need to be present at the hospital. The team can be helpful to identify supports within the community to assist with child-care, meals, transportation, or other needs, particularly when the hospitalization is prolonged. An underused resource perhaps may be the team's ability to provide support and partnership to the medical team. Their insight helps to maintain continuity of care when multiple services are involved, and these services continue over many years. The palliative care team also has a wealth of knowledge to convey to assist the health care team to understand the impact of chronic illness on a child and family, use of various medications and nonpharmacological interventions for symptom relief, and how to navigate the moral or ethical concerns that come with caring for children with medical complexity.

SUMMARY

Our children's hospitals are filled with children who would not have survived decades ago. Children who died years ago, are now living with congenital conditions, sequelae of premature birth, complications of birth, and resultant chronic medical conditions. We have an opportunity to make life with these conditions have quality and meaning by openly discussing what quality looks like, identifying interventions that enhance quality and those that do not provide benefit. As a health care team, we need to engage with parents and patients to provide care that is consistent with identified goals and values and be comfortable not offering or providing interventions that are not consistent with identified values. We need to assist families in continuing to explore their thoughts over time as the underlying disease progresses or the availability of treatment changes.

CLINICS CARE POINTS

- Prenatal palliative care can assist parents make decisions when a life-threatening diagnosis is presented or a disease-modifying treatment for a chronic condition no longer provides benefit.
- There are many examples of novel therapies that are changing the way we look at disease.
- Anticipatory guidance can be provided to families who need help exploring goals of care as disease progresses.
- Clinical information that care teams may consider upsetting is the information parents need to make effective decisions about their child's care.
- Parents who are unable to describe quality of life for their child tend to choose intense and invasive interventions that mat cause suffering near the end of life.

DISCLOSURE

The author has nothing to disclose.

REFERENCES

1. Burns KH, Casey PH, Lyle RE, et al. Increasing prevalence of medically complex children in U.S. hospitals. Pediatrics 2010;126(4):638–46.
2. O'Keefe S, Maddux AB, Bennett KS, et al. Variation in pediatric palliative care allocation among critically ill children in the United States. Pediatr Crit Care Med 2021;22(5):462–73.
3. Grunauer M, Mikesell C. A review of the integrated mode of care: an opportunity to respond to extensive palliative care needs in pediatric intensive care units in under-resourced settings. Front Pediatr 2018;6:3. Available at: https://www.frontiersin.org/articles/10.3389/fped.2018.00003/full. Accessed July 15, 2021.
4. Hays RM, Valentine J, Haynes G, et al. The seattle pediatric palliative care Project: Effects on family satisfaction and health-related quality of life. J Palliat Med 2006;9:716–28.
5. Frazier A, Frazier H, Warren NA. A discussion of family-centered care within the pediatric intensive care unit. Crit Care Nurs Q 2009;33:82–6.
6. Truog RD, Meyer EC, Burns JP. Toward interventions to improve end-of-life care in the pediatric intensive care unit. Crit Care Med 2006;34(Suppl. 11):S373–9.
7. Meyer EC, Ritzholz MD, Burns JP, et al. Improving the quality of end-of life care in the pediatric intensive care unit: parents' priorities and recommendations. Pediatrics 2006;117(3):649–57.

8. Aslakson R, Curtis JR, Nelson JE. The changing role of palliative care in the ICU. Crit Care Med 2014;42(11):2418–28.

9. Mack JW, Hilden JM, Watterson J, et al. Parent and physician perspectives on quality of care at the end of life in children with cancer. J Clin Oncol 2005;23: 9155–61.

10. World Health Organization. Palliative care. 2010. Available at: http://www.who.int/cancer/palliative/en. Accessed July 15, 2021.

11. Feudtner C, Kang TI, Hexem KR, et al. Pediatric palliative care patients: a prospective multi-center cohort study. Pediatrics 2011;127:1094–101.

12. Hauer J, Poplack DG, Armsby C. Pediatric palliative care. UpToDate®. 2021. Available at. www.uptodate.com. Accessed July 15, 2021.

13. Oskoui M, Darras BT, DeVivo DC. Chapter 1- Spinal muscular atrophy: 125 years later and on the verge of a cure. Spinal Muscular Atrophy. Available at: https://wwwsciencedirect.com/science/article/pii/B978012803685300001X. Accessed July 15, 2021.

14. Mack JW, Wolfe J, Cook EF, et al. Hope and prognostic disclosure. J Clin Oncol 2007;25:5636.

15. Mack JW, Wolfe J, Grier HE, et al. Communications about prognosis between parents and physicians of children with cancer: parent preferences and the impact of prognostic information. J Clin Oncol 2006;24:5265.

16. Wolfe J, Klar N, Grier HE, et al. Understanding of prognosis among parents of children who died of cancer: impact on treatment goals and integration of palliative care. JAMA 2000;284:2469.

17. Weeks JC, Cook EF, O'Day SJ, et al. Relationship between cancer patients' predictions of prognosis and their treatment preferences. JAMA 1998;279:1709.

18. Wolfe J, Grier HE, Klar N, et al. Symptoms and suffering at the end of life in children with cancer. N Engl J Med 2000;342:326.

19. Drake R, Frost J, Collins JJ. The symptoms of dying children. J Pain Symptom Manage 2003;26:594.

20. Hunt A, Burne R. Medical and nursing problems of children with neurodegenerative disease. Palliat Med 1995;9:19.

Minority Populations and the Use of Palliative Care

Dorothy N. Pierce, DNP, RN, NP-C, CRN, CBCN, CRNI, CLT

KEYWORDS

- Minority populations • Health disparities • Palliative care • Culture • Spirituality
- Patient education

KEY POINTS

- Palliative care (PC) starts when a patient is diagnosed with a life-threatening disease. Health disparities continue for an array of nationalities but are markedly influenced by inequities.
- PC is a path that improves the quality of life of patients afflicted with life-threatening conditions through prevention, early recognition, and treatment of physical, psychosocial, and spiritual predicaments.
- Palliative radiotherapy is perceived to be part of the multidisciplinary team that aims to slow disease progression or symptoms control and alleviate patient suffering.

Racial disparities exist, and outcomes arise from inequities at many levels in the US health care system, including cancer screening, timely diagnosis, and treatment to palliative and end-of-life (EOL) care. As a result, markedly minority populations in the United States continue to forbear a disproportionate burden of disease, risk factors, unmet health care needs, and other health conditions.[1] PC should be an essential component in managing minority populations, specifically those with chronic diseases and advanced cancer, precisely when symptom management becomes a challenge.[2] Notably, the appropriate and timely symptom interventions, patient education, and side-effect management may help minimize emergency department (ED) visits and intensive care hospitalizations while maximizing patients' function.[2] Despite the growth in PC availability over 20 years, it has gained significant acceptance in our health care system for people with socioeconomic means and resources but not for the minority populations.[3,4] Persist in the United States, distinctively, it has been documented that cancer care disparities, owing to racial or ethnic bias, literacy level, socioeconomic status, health insurance coverage, and other factors.[5] Certain minority populations diagnosed with advanced disease, particularly the Hispanics, the homeless, and African Americans (AA), disproportionately experienced inequities compared

Radiation Oncology, Rutgers Cancer Institute of New Jersey, 195 Little Albany Street, New Brunswick, NJ 08903, USA
E-mail address: piercedn@cinj.rutgers.edu

Crit Care Nurs Clin N Am 34 (2022) 19–29
https://doi.org/10.1016/j.cnc.2021.11.002
0899-5885/22/© 2021 Elsevier Inc. All rights reserved.

with other groups in the US population.[3,6] This article addresses the minority populations and PC use, emphasizing people of color and the homeless. How can the PC team help decrease these disparities to benefit patients and their caregivers in the minority communities?

HISTORY

Today, PC has grown exponentially in the United States and is available within extended-care facilities, outpatient clinics, home care settings, and many inpatient hospital settings.[7] In particular, state-by-state report card data on access to PC, with 72% of US hospitals (with 50 or more beds) and 94% of large hospitals (with 300 or more beds), report a PC team.[8] Public hospitals, which care for approximately 44 million patients who are disproportionately minorities, Medicaid beneficiaries, the uninsured, or those living in disadvantaged communities, are less likely to receive PC services, with only 60% reporting a PC team.[8]

Inpatient consultations have identified unrecognized symptoms and unmet needs associated with fewer intensive care and intensive care unit deaths.[9] The lack of access to palliative consultations results in fewer PC benefits to rural and minority patients.[9] It has been documented that "by 2044, the people of color will comprise more than 50% of the population. In addition, by 2060, 20% of Americans are projected to be foreign-born and individuals who identify themselves as belonging to two or more races."[7] Most importantly, historical and social factors, including slavery, racism, medical experimentation, and exploitation, as well as ongoing racism and microaggressions, have left a deep-seated legacy of distrust in the AA community.

In 1965, during the civil rights evolution, Dr Martin Luther King Jr addressed health disparities. He said that "of all the forms of inequality, injustice in health is the most shocking and the most inhuman because it often results in physical death."[10]

IMPORTANT DEFINITIONS

The Centers for Disease Control and Prevention (CDC) defines racial and ethnic minority populations to include Hispanics or Latinos, Native Hawaiians, Asian Americans, black or AA, Pacific Islanders, American Indians, and Alaska Natives.[11] These groups are individuals that have experienced barriers owing to their racial or ethnic class, religion, socioeconomic status, gender, age, mental health, cognitive, sensory, or physical disability, sexual orientation, or geographic location, which historically have been linked to discrimination or exclusion.[12] In this case, social determinants of health (SDoH) must be seriously taken into consideration. Essentially, in the United States, one of the most significant challenges in reducing the profound disparity in the health status of its racial and ethnic minority, rural, low-income, and other underserved population is paramount.[13] This means removing obstacles to health, such as poverty, discrimination, and their consequences, including powerlessness and lack of access to health care.[14] Steinhauser and colleagues[15] mentioned that PC spiritually is often operationalized related to diverse spiritual or religious beliefs, rituals, practices, coping, distress, relationship with the transcendent, sense of meaning, or life purpose. **Box 1** highlights the most important definitions.[3,4,12,14,16–19]

BACKGROUND

It has been documented that scientific and technological inventions have enriched the health of the US population overall.[13] Still, there are concerns about inequities

Box 1
Important definitions addressing minority disparities

- Health disparities: Differences in health outcomes that are intricately linked with social, economic, and environmental disadvantage are driven by the social conditions in which individuals live, learn, work, and play.

- Social determinants of health: The conditions in which people are born, grow, work, live, and age, and the broader set of forces and systems shaping the needs of daily life.

- Disparities: The ability of any person to have equal and just opportunities to maintain and improve their health.

- Social inequality: Social disadvantage refers to the unfavorable social, economic, or political conditions that some groups systematically experience based on their relative position in social hierarchies.

- Palliative care: An interdisciplinary approach of care used to improve the quality of life for patients and families living with and dying from advanced disease through the prevention and relief of symptoms by the impeccable assessment and management of pain and other problems, physical, psychosocial, and spiritual.[15]

- Culture: The learned and shared behavior of a community of interacting human beings.

- Cultural competency: Ability to interact effectively with people of different cultures.

- Spiritually: The core of the whole person PC.

Data from Refs.[3,4,12,14,16–18]

because of systemic racism, making it less likely that members of racial and ethnic minority groups can benefit.[7,13]

Elements affiliated with this phenomenon include economic and social factors that frame a person's daily life, consequently, SDoH. The CDC highlighted that "unequal access to care and unequal treatment of persons who receive care are key determinants of racial, ethnic disparities in health care."[1] Mainly, research has shown that individuals working with the homeless have doubts about whether the homeless have equal access to quality PC.[6] Evidence-based data showed that people experiencing homelessness often procrastinate on how their life will end. The diversity and complexity of health problems and the needs in different areas of life pose challenges to access favorable PC.[6] Similarly, such care is less widely available to people experiencing homelessness.[6]

At-risk patients with advanced disease will capitulate to their condition eventually. Regrettably, these patients remain clueless about their illness and demise because of a lack of pertinent communication regarding their prognosis. **Fig. 1** illustrates the interconnectedness of the 4 phases of PC of patients with advanced disease. PC does not mean denial, referral to treatment delivery, standard curative care and euthanasia, or physician-assisted suicide. Research studies show that PC decreases symptom burden, improves the quality of life, and enhances patient and caregiver satisfaction.[4]

PC's goal is to assist individuals with advanced health concerns, cancer, including symptoms management, for example, pain control, to improve quality of life for both patient and family.[20] PC should be sought out earlier in the disease journey and can be provided in conjunction with curative intent or interventions that aim to minimize the symptoms related to the disease process.[20] Early evidence-based data determined that despite the significant gains that have been made toward the Institute of Medicine quality recommendations, achieving equity has remained ambiguous and gleans

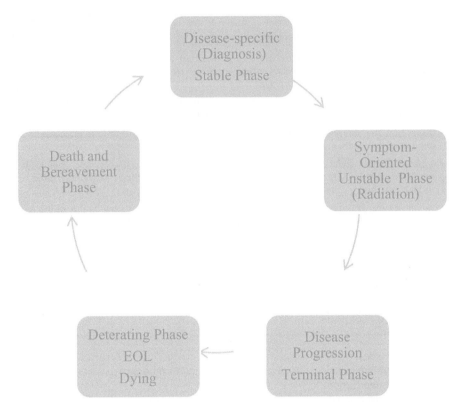

Fig. 1. Goal: coordinating complementary care across disease trajectory (outpatient and inpatient), either to rehabilitation or through death. (*Image courtesy of* Dorothy N. Pierce. Used with permission.)

convincingly less attention than the others.[7] Most existing studies highlight that equity is the principle that quality of care should not vary based on patient characteristics, such as race or ethnicity.[7] Nevertheless, racial and ethnic disparities in quality of care contribute to inequalities in health outcomes in the United States among the minority populations.[4]

MINORITY POPULATION UNDERUTILIZATION OF PALLIATIVE SERVICES

PC is specialized medical care for people with severe illness, is appropriate at any stage in severe disease, and can be provided to patients together with standard treatment.[1,21] Ultimately, PC care focuses on providing patients relief from symptoms, pain, stress, and distress of a severe illness. For instance, radiation therapy (RT) is an essential component of multidisciplinary supportive care (see Case Presentation for PC management). Pain and discomfort are the exclusive most prevalent symptoms for patients receiving palliative radiation. It has been documented that AA experience high-cost, low-quality care, described by untreated pain, avoidable hospitalizations, and poor communication with providers, receiving care unpredictable with their desires.[22] Moreover, Dharmarajan and colleagues[21] illuminated that the main barriers to receiving palliative radiation are related to underreferral. Some reasons patients are not referred to radiation oncology are incomplete knowledge about the utility of radiation as a potential pain management option.[21] PC has been particularly underutilized by AA and Latino older adults and those who live in low-income, medically underserved areas.[23] There is an overall lack of participation by black patients in all programs related to EOL care; this includes aid in dying, and the authors consider this lack a health care disparity.[3,23]

Some minority groups generally disagree in statements, "black people prefer more aggressive treatment at EOL."[3] This can be translated as a form of discrimination and stereotyping of a specific group. Griggs[3] proposes that black, Native American, and Alaskan Native patients are less likely to receive outpatient PC services, and therefore, inpatient admission is primarily sought by minorities. Amazingly, the investigator mentioned that little is known about referral decoration and uptake of outpatient PC among Hispanic or Asian populations in the United States.[3]

BARRIERS TO UTILIZATION OF MINORITY PALLIATIVE CARE

Factors contributing to the disparities in minorities accessing PC are not well documented; nevertheless, the primary purpose of PC is proper management of physical and psychosocial distress.[24] The research found that early reports showed striking disparities among blacks, and emerging data on race and ethnicity have uncovered similar inequities in Latinos and Native Americans.[24] Martinez and colleagues[24] articulated that historically Latinos have had lower access to health care, including cancer screening and treatment, because of lack of insurance and inadequate insurance coverage.

Moreover, research data illuminated that disparities affecting diverse populations reveal poverty.[23] Gardner and colleagues[23] particularly highlighted a research study that explored barriers to PC in 5 urban communities and found that minority stress, feelings of disempowerment, and lack of community supports posed further barriers to accessing PC services.

Cultural beliefs and treatment preferences are barriers to the use of PC in marginalized groups.[9] For instance, research among AA mentioned that spiritual and religious beliefs may conflict with PC's goals, and mistrust of the health care system owing to past injustices and the ongoing disparities lead to concerns about forgoing curative care.[9] Other cultural beliefs that may present a barrier to using PC include fewer positive attitudes toward disclosing terminal illness.[9] Culture is paramount; it shapes how individuals make meaning out of condition, suffering, and dying, and it decidedly influences people's resources to diagnosis, illness, and treatment preferences.[9] Surprisingly, the investigators emphasized that a lack of sensitivity to cultural differences may compromise EOL care for minority patients.[9]

Remarkably, the triple threat of rural geography, racial inequalities, and older age hampers access to high-quality PC for rural Americans.[9] Elk and colleagues[9] make visible, even when palliative and hospice services are available. Compared with whites, AA are more likely to receive medically ineffective, poor-quality, high-cost care because of general mistrust of health care providers.[9] The fragmented health care system is customarily insensitive to cultural differences that can assist with treatment choices.[9] Even though there has been proven effectiveness, numerous studies have shown that AA underutilize palliative and hospice care.[9] Elk and colleagues[9] suggested that this inequality is the lack of exposure to hospice or PC information and possibly differences in values for EOL care.

PC and EOL care have been entrenched in white middle-class cultural and religious values.[9] Its hugely different frame of reference, value system, and life experience compared with many AA where middle-class whites may accentuate individual choice. In addition, AA values support family-centered decision making.[9] Steinhauser and colleagues[15] mentioned that religious factors might play a role in influencing differences in EOL outcomes.[15] The investigators noted that AA and Latino are the largest racial, ethnic minority groups in the United States and are typically more religious and receive more aggressive EOL intervention than white patients. The investigators mentioned that "spirituality is a dynamic and intrinsic aspect to humanity through, which persons seek ultimate meaning, purpose, and transcendence, and experience relationship to self, family, others, community, society, nature and the significant or sacred."[15]

Remarkably, the investigators highlighted that spirituality is communicated through beliefs, values, traditions, and practices.[15] Strikingly, in the AA community, faith, spiritual beliefs, and guidance of a spiritual leader are very meaningful, especially as they cope with illness and make treatment decisions.[9] It has been documented that AA and Latino patients have more significant endorsement of religious beliefs about medical care and religious coping.[15] Research has shown that AA and whites were disassociated in their perceptions of racial equality and actual gaps. Inequality is even more strongly felt in the Southern States, where slavery was promoted.[9]

Another study found that AA are more likely than other racial groups to believe that physicians did not care about them as individuals and were less likely to trust their judgment and personal competence.[9,15] Organizational barriers to PC by racial and ethnic minorities include the absence of minority physicians, nurses, and other staff and community outreach to diverse communities. Ghesquiere and colleagues[4] noted critical barriers to PC utilization because it is mainly provided on an inpatient basis. After all, few outpatients or community-based PC services exist. The lack of familiarity among patients as to the meaning of PC is often confused with hospice care. Outpatient PC services remain underutilized. Research has shown that only 8% to 18% of patients receive PC care consultation more than 30 days before death.[25]

PHYSICIAN AND NURSES INFLUENCE ON MINORITY PALLIATIVE CARE

PC nurses should realize that the degree to which caregiving is a cultural obligation may influence seeking support.[26] PC is a multilayered artistic concept. Culture influences one's thinking and behavior.[26] Six and colleagues[26] notably determined a strong indication for cultural differences in PC regarding autonomy, attitudes toward and expression of pain, and control over death. For example, a direct influence of cultural values and norms on health decisions are the religious groups that prefer to put their fate in the hands of God and do not wish medical intervention. For physicians and nurses to provide PC to the culturally diverse minority population, the individual needs to exhibit knowledge, skills, patience, trust, compassion, honesty, and, most importantly, communication.[26] The ability to communicate well is essential for quality patient care.[27] It has been associated with higher patient satisfaction, better patient outcomes, less patient anxiety, better adherence to treatments, and better care at the EOL.[26] Six and colleagues[26] illuminated that to develop cultural competence in PC, it is crucial to recognize that one's own culture also merits enlightened examination. It is far from a neutral background against which other cultures may measure.

IMPROVING ACCESS TO MINORITY PALLIATIVE CARE

These are recommendations on improving access to PC for at-risk minority patients.[28] Essentially, a series of organizational changes are needed to end racial disparities; until every patient has equal access to treatment facilities and affordable health care, differences will continue to be seen.[28] Theoretically, developing culturally competent educational materials and improving health literacy may improve access for these groups.[28] Importantly, data collection is significant, leading to policy change for these minority groups.[28] Other areas to address are implementing PC navigators and social support to address disparities in the PC setting.[28] Finally, everyone should have access to health care undeniably, if they are burdened financially.[28] This work should consider the full spectrum of racial and ethnic groups across diagnoses and care settings.[28]

Notably, health care system efforts to reduce disparities should target patients, providers, communities, and health policy and ensure that new models of care accommodate the range of needs and preferences of a rapidly growing racially and ethnically diverse population.[29] Racial and ethnic disparities occur in every health care system, for example, the patient, the provider, and the health care system.[29] For example, structural racism and discrimination are alive and well in the US health care system, limiting opportunities to their minority employees, and cannot be discounted.[29] Wheeler and Bryant[29] mentioned that providers, although well meaning, are subject to implicit biases that can negatively impact interactions with minority patients and contribute to disparities. What is not known is the extent of the discrimination in the health care system.[29]

In addition, for example, at an urban health care system that would benefit from minority trained PC health care professionals, which does not currently reflect the diversity of the population. Employees often experience structural racism from other colleagues; frankly, racial discrimination within the system limits opportunity resources linked to substantial health disparities.[9] Similarly, the opportunity to complete the PC internship training to a minority employee was denied, resulting in differences and unequal access to work-related resources. This situation was an opportunity for a minority employee clinician to deliver care to the at-risk patients at the facility for the patient population served, which would add merit personally and professionally.

Another vital aspect of PC is the lack of education. According to Thompson and colleagues,[30] patients need education about PC services before they can be used. The investigators emphasized that mobile applications have been a practical option and convenient and efficient way to provide education. In addition, Thompson and colleagues[30] illuminated that the use of educational apps may lead to more open discussions among patients, family, and providers about PC and potentially lead to earlier referrals.[30] The literature shows that little research has been done at the patient level regarding integrating further PC services into their care.[30]

CASE PRESENTATION

Offering palliative RT is an essential, interprofessional approach to cancer care for all patients. The principal goal of RT is to eradicate or control tumor cells while minimizing toxicity to the surrounding normal tissues. RT also can be given to achieve cure; however, if a treatment is not realistic, RT can be provided to control disease progression. Moreover, RT can be administered during the terminal stage of cancer for palliative relief of pain caused by bone metastasis, obstruction caused by tumor progression, or uncontrolled bleeding resulting from tumor invasion of the vascular system.

Case A

C.R. is a 79-year-old man admitted with bilateral leg weakness, difficulty walking, and back pain. The patient has a history of well-differentiated invasive squamous cell carcinoma. Radiological evidence showed a large lytic destructive, pathologic fracture at T3 along with metastatic invasion, severe central canal stenosis, and compression of

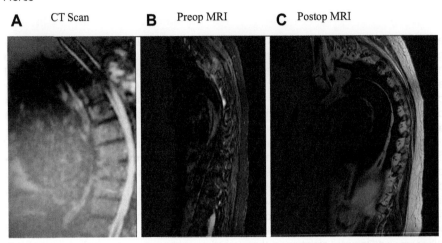

Fig. 2. MRI: thoracic spine scan. (*A*) CT: thoracic spine scan shows a malignant soft tissue mass involving lateral displacement and compression of the spinal cord. (*B*) MRI: large destructive mass involving the T2 and T3 posterior producing severe central canal stenosis and compression of the bilateral T2 nerve roots and left T3 nerve root. Mild cord edema at T3. (*C*) MRI: postsurgical intervention T2 and T3 for resection of destructive lesion with resolution of cord compression and improving cord edema at the T3 level. Postop, postoperative; Preop, preoperative. (*Image courtesy of* Dorothy N. Pierce. Used with permission.)

the bilateral T2 nerve roots and left T3 nerve root. The patient underwent T2 and T3 laminectomy for resection, recovered reasonably well, and received palliative RT to the region for residual disease, receiving a dose of 30 Gy in 10 fractions (**Fig. 2**).

Case B

J.R. is a 60-year-old man admitted to an ED with a sudden onset of bilateral lower-extremities weakness, numbness, and dyspnea. Radiologic evidence showed diffuse bony metastases, likely spinal cord compression, large right lung lesion, and solitary brain metastasis. Physical examination revealed an extensive injury to the spinal cord at the level of the tumor with minimal residual function, bilateral lower extremities, and decreased respiratory dysfunction secondary to bronchus obstruction. Surgery is the treatment of choice to decompress the spine to improve function. However, given the patient's neurologic and pulmonary function, the patient was deemed a poor surgical candidate.

Bone biopsy was performed to obtain histologic confirmation, and pathology revealed metastatic disease consistent with the pulmonary primary. PC consultation was requested for assistance with determining the goals of care and additional support.

Given that surgical intervention was deemed impossible, J.R. opted for palliative radiotherapy to 30 Gy in 10 fractions. Metastatic spinal cord compression (MSCC) is a prevalent problem of metastatic malignancies, and MSCC is an oncological emergency that must be diagnosed and treated early. The treatment is performed to prevent MSCC correlated morbidity, which could cause loss of mobility, sphincter control, and pain. After histologic and radiological affirmation, the standard treatment is radiotherapy. Exceptions are patients with gross spinal instability and compression, secondary to bone impingement, which require surgery, as this patient from the case presentation.

SUMMARY

Although multiple factors are known to affect health care disparities, access to a receipt of relevant PC offered to minority communities may be an attainable goal to ensure equal access to quality care.[29] Despite PC availability and improvements in access to mostly inpatient PC for racial and ethnic minorities, there is detritus room for improvements to enhance disparities at the organizational level.[29] The elimination of racial-ethnic differences in health status will require essential changes in how health care is delivered and financed in the United States.[1] Research must be implemented to explore disparity utilization and quality of PC, understand the SDoH disparities, and develop interventions to reduce disparities and improve the care of seriously ill minorities. Attempts to reduce disparities should include targeting strategies at the local level, advocacy, community empowerment, patients, providers, health systems, and health policy to ensure the range of demand and choices of a growing racially and ethnically diverse populations in the United States.

CLINICS CARE POINTS

- The goal of palliative care is to boost quality of life.
- Palliative care comprises care provided to patients anywhere during the illness journey from diagnosis to cure or death to alleviate illness-related anguish.
- All physicians have the burden of discussing end-of-life opinions before catastrophe along a patient illness trajectory before catastrophe with all patients with life-threatening illnesses.
- The interdisciplinary team is imperative, and radiation oncology offers a decisive opportunity to address care, prognosis, and EOL treatment preferences with patients and families.
- Communication with patients and families is paramount for quality patient care.

DISCLOSURE

None.

REFERENCES

1. Center for Disease Control and Prevention. Health disparities experienced by racial ethnic minority populations. Available at: http://www.cdc.gov. [Accessed 2 July 2021].
2. Hui D, Hannon B, Zimmermann C, et al. Improving patient and caregiver outcomes in oncology: team-based, timely, and targeted palliative care. CA Cancer J Clin 2018;68(5):356–76.
3. Griggs JJ. Disparities in palliative care in patients with cancer. J Clin Oncol 2020; 38(9):974–9.
4. Ghesquiere A, Gardner D, McAfee C, et al. Development of a community-based palliative screening tool for underserved older adults with chronic illness. Am J Hosp Palliat Care 2018;35(7):929–37.
5. Oyer A, Smeltzer MP, Kramar A, et al. Equity-driven approaches to optimizing cancer care coordination and reducing care delivery disparities in underserved patient populations in the United States. J Clin Oncol 2021;17(5):215–8. https://doi.org/10.1200/op.20.00895.
6. De Veer AJE, Stringer B, Van Meijel B, et al. Access to palliative care for homeless people: complex lives, complex care. Biomed Cent Palliat Care 2018; 17(119):1–11.
7. Betancourt JR, Tan-McGrory A, Flores E. Racial and ethnic disparities in radiology: a call to action. J Am Coll Radiol 2019;16:547–53.

8. Center to Advance Palliative Care. American's care of serious illness. A state-by-state report card on access to palliative care in our nation's hospital, 2019. Available at: https://reportcard.capc.org. [Accessed 25 May 2021].

9. Elk R, Emanuel L, Hauser J, et al. Developing and testing the feasibility of a culturally based tele-palliative care consul based on the cultural values and preferences of southern, rural African American and white community members: a program by and for the community. Health Equity 2020;4(1):52–83.

10. Galarneau C. Getting King's words right. J Health Care Poor Underserved 2018; 29(1):5–9.

11. Fiscella K, Sanders M. Racial and ethnic disparities in the quality of health care. Annu Rev Public Health 2016;37:375–94.

12. Healthy people 2020. Disparities. Available at: https://www.healthypeople.gov/2020/about/foundation-health-measures/Disparities. Accessed June 27, 2021.

13. National Institute on Minority Health and Health Disparities. Available at: https://www.nimhd.nih.gov. [Accessed 7 July 2021].

14. Braveman P, Arkin E, Orleans T. What is health equity. Robert Wood Johnson Foundation; 2017. Available at: https://www.rwj.org/en/library/research%20/2017/05/what-is-health-equity-html. [Accessed 27 June 2021].

15. Steinhauser KE, Fitchett G, Handzo GF, et al. State of science of spirituality and palliative care research part 1: definitions, measurement, and outcomes. J Pain Symptom Manage 2017;54(3):428–39.

16. Phillips J, Richard A, Mayer KN, et al. Integrating social determinants of health into nursing practice: nurses' perspectives. J Nurs Scholarsh 2020;52(5): 497–505.

17. Kuebler K, Acker KA, Froelich SD. Overview. In: Kuebler K, editor. Integration of palliative care in chronic conditions: an interdisciplinary approach. Pittsburgh (PA): Oncology Nursing Society; 2017. p. 1–12.

18. Center for Disease Control and Prevention. Cultural and diversity considerations. Available at: www.cdc.gov/tb/education/skillscourse/day2/culture-and-diversity-considerations_final.pptx. [Accessed 2 July 2021].

19. Campos-Castillo C, Anthony D. Racial and ethnic differences in self-reported telehealth use during the COVID-19 pandemic: a secondary analysis of a US survey of internet users from late March. J Am Med Inform Assoc 2021;28(1):119–25.

20. Bazargan M, Bazargan-Hejazi S. Disparities in palliative and hospice care and completion of advance care planning and directives among non-Hispanic blacks: a scoping review of recent literature. Am J Hosp Palliat Med 2021;38(6):688–718.

21. Dharmarajan KV, Rich SE, Johnstone CA. Top 10 tips palliative care clinicians should know about radiation oncology. J Palliat Med 2018;21(3):383–8.

22. Ejem DB, Barrett N, Rhodes RL. Reducing disparities in the quality of palliative care for older African Americans through improved advance care planning: study design and protocol. J Palliat Med 2019;22(S1). S-90-S-100.

23. Gardner DS, Parikh NS, Villanueva CH. Assessing the palliative care needs and service use of diverse older adults in an urban medically underserved community. Ann Palliat Med 2019;8(5):769–74.

24. Martinez ME, Nodora JN, Carvajal-Carmona LG. The dual pandemic of COVID-19 and systemic inequities in US Latino communities. Cancer 2021;127:1548–50.

25. Graul A, Haggerty A, Stickley C. Effect of patient education on palliative care knowledge and acceptability of outpatient palliative care services among gynecologic oncology patients: a randomized controlled trial. Gynecol Oncol 2020; 156:482–7.

26. Six S, Bilsen J, Deschepper R. Dealing with cultural diversity in palliative care. Br Med J Support Palliat Care 2020;0:1–5.
27. Goswami P. Advance care planning and end-of-life communications: practical tips for oncology advanced practitioners. J Adv Pract Oncol 2021;12(1):89–95.
28. Digiulio S. Oncologists raise alarm about health inequities in US Latino communities. Oncology Times 2021;43(12):12.
29. Wheeler SM, Bryant AS. Racial and ethnic disparities in health and healthcare. Obstet Gynecol Clin North Am 2017;44:1–11.
30. Thompson SL, Ward C, Galanos A. Impact of a palliative care education module in patients with heart disease. Am J Hosp Palliat Med 2020;37(12):1016–21.

A Scoping Review of the Experiences of Adolescents and Young Adults in the ICU, Their Family Members, and Their Health Care Team

Natalie S. McAndrew, PhD, RN, ACNS-BC, CCRN-K[a,b,*],
Jeanne M. Erickson, PhD, RN[a], Jill Guttormson, PhD, RN[c],
Alexandria Bear, MD[d], Sean Marks, MD[d], Jayshil Patel, MD[e],
Eric S. Harding, MLS[f]

KEYWORDS

- Adolescents • Young adults • Intensive care unit • Experiences • Family • Parents

KEY POINTS

- Adolescents and young adults (AYAs) with critical illness and their caregivers may have distinct needs and distress that stem from their developmental life stage.
- Evidence about the experiences of AYAs in the ICU is limited, and specific literature about young adults in the ICU was nearly nonexistent.
- Health care professionals need to involve AYAs and their family members in decision making and consider ways to offer developmentally tailored resources in the ICU.
- There are opportunities to improve serious illness communication skills and advance care planning for AYAs who require ICU care.

[a] University of Wisconsin-Milwaukee, College of Nursing, 1921 East Hartford Avenue, Milwaukee, WI 53211, USA; [b] Froedtert & the Medical College of Wisconsin Froedtert Hospital, 9200 West Wisconsin Avenue, Milwaukee, WI 53226, USA; [c] Marquette University, College of Nursing, PO Box 1881, Milwaukee, WI 53201, USA; [d] Department of Medicine, Division of Geriatric and Palliative Medicine, Medical College of Wisconsin, 9200 W. Wisconsin Avenue, Milwaukee, WI 53226, USA; [e] Department of Medicine, Division of Pulmonary, Critical Care and Sleep Medicine, Medical College of Wisconsin, 9200 W. Wisconsin Avenue, Milwaukee, WI 53226, USA; [f] Medical College of Wisconsin Libraries, 8701 Watertown Plank Road, Milwaukee, WI 53226, USA
* Corresponding author. University of Wisconsin-Milwaukee, College of Nursing, 1921 East Hartford Avenue, Milwaukee, WI 53211.
E-mail address: mcandre3@uwm.edu

Crit Care Nurs Clin N Am 34 (2022) 31–55
https://doi.org/10.1016/j.cnc.2021.11.003
0899-5885/22/© 2021 Elsevier Inc. All rights reserved.

INTRODUCTION

Adolescent and young adult (AYA) is a term that has emerged in health care to specify a unique developmental period and population. AYAs are in a transitional period between childhood and mature adulthood, resulting in specific health care needs and experiences that are distinct from younger children and older adults. Health care providers are challenged to provide age-specific care for AYAs and their families across specialties to improve AYAs' health outcomes. Although there is no consensus about the age parameters for AYAs, the broadest definition defines AYAs as individuals between the ages of 15 years old and 39 years old.[1]

Adolescence/young adulthood is a dynamic period of development, with transitional milestones related to becoming independent from parents, advancing toward career and work goals, choosing life partners, and establishing families of their own.[2] This vulnerable period also is characterized by risk-taking behaviors and feelings of invincibility.[3] Age-related health disparities are evident in this population due to greater violence and injury, being uninsured, not having a primary care provider, and delays in seeking health care, often leading to poorer health care outcomes.[4] The leading causes of morbidity and mortality in this age group include unintentional injury, homicide, suicide, cancer, and heart disease.[5]

ICU admissions for AYAs are not uncommon and may be due to injury, malignancy, substance abuse, or exacerbations and complications related to pediatric-onset chronic illnesses.[6] AYAs, depending on their age, may be cared for in either an adult ICU or pediatric ICU. In a recent search of the Vizient Clinical Database pre-COVID-19, the authors found that AYAs (individuals younger than 39 years old) account for approximately 15.3% of admissions to adult ICUs.[7] In adult ICUs, a majority of patients are 50 years or older,[8] whereas in a pediatric ICU, a majority of patients are under 10 years of age.[9] The developmental and supportive needs of AYAs differ from those of the populations typically served in adult and pediatric ICUs.

The limited AYA-related critical care research suggests some important trends in AYA ICU care.[6,10] In 1 study that examined AYA ICU admissions, in comparison to older adults, AYA patients more often were male, more often were African American/black, and had shorter median lengths of stays that were largely related to risk-taking behaviors and pediatric chronic illness.[6] In a sample of 705 AYA patients with cancer (ages 15–29 years), 21% had an ICU stay, 75% received high-intensity end-of-life care, 65% died in an acute care setting, and only 23% received hospice care.[11] The ICU providers may offer AYA patients aggressive ICU care based on their assumption that these younger patients would benefit from life-saving and sustaining treatments.[12]

To fully understand the needs and improve care of the AYA population during an ICU stay, the experiences of the ICU team caring for AYAs also must be comprehended. Caring for an adolescent or young adult in a pediatric ICU may be challenging for a health care professional who works more commonly with younger children. Similarly, caring for an AYA in an adult ICU may pose challenges to health care professionals who are accustomed to working with older adults. ICU clinicians report more distress when caring for AYAs than when caring for critically ill children or adults.[13] Efforts to increase health care professionals' knowledge and awareness of the unique needs of AYA populations could improve the clinical practice of those caring for AYAs in both pediatric KICU and adult ICU settings. The authors' research team held in-depth discussions about their clinical experiences with AYAs in the ICU setting. To frame this scoping review, the authors describe a case of an AYA patient that illustrates unique critical illness challenges in this population. Some details of this case have been changed to protect the patient's anonymity.

EXEMPLAR CASE

Violet, 28 years old, was admitted to the adult ICU and experienced ventilator-dependent chronic respiratory failure, refractory pain, anxiety, delirium, multisystem organ failure, and malnutrition. Despite escalation of life-prolonging interventions, Violet experienced progressive medical decline over 9 months and ultimately died from complications of her underlying illness. Violet was not married, had no designated health care proxy, and had no advanced directive. Violet voiced her desire to live for her young children, and, when she was given options, chose life-supportive interventions. Because Violet had not designated a health care power of attorney (HCPOA), it was unclear whether the appropriate surrogate decision maker (SDM) should be her mother (Donna) or her partner, the father of her young children. Although Violet was not close to her mother, as her condition worsened, Donna stepped in and became her sole decision maker. The team had concerns about Donna's well-being and her ability to cope with her daughter's serious illness and imminent death. There was ongoing conflict among the health care team about changing goals of care to prevent unnecessary suffering. The team experienced moral distress about how Violet's care unfolded, and this distress was compounded by her young age.

As the research team reconsidered Violet's case, the authors wondered if unique factors, such as her young adult status and lack of appointed SDM, may have contributed to our concerns about her suffering and long length of stay in the ICU. Did the authors have different expectations of recovery for this young adult patient versus an older adult with comorbidities? Are there differences in the authors' experiences as health care professionals caring for younger patients versus older patients? Did the authors meet the needs of this young adult patient and her parent? What about her young children, significant other, and extended family members and friends? These lingering questions led the team to explore through a scoping review what is known about the serious illness experiences of the adolescent and young adult population in the ICU setting from the perspective of 3 key stakeholders: patients, family members, and health care professionals.

There have been multiple calls to address the palliative care needs of AYAs.[14,15] Given gaps in the integration of palliative care in critical care environments for both pediatric ICUs and adult-focused ICUs, however, studying the experiences of AYAs in ICUs, their family members, and their ICU team may uncover opportunities to better address the developmental needs of AYAs with serious illnesses. Therefore, the purpose of our scoping review iss to describe the extent, range, and nature of existing literature pertaining to AYA experiences in the ICU setting and identify key gaps to guide future research specific to this population and setting.

METHODS

A scoping review is the method of choice when a topic has not previously been reviewed extensively.[16] This scoping review was guided by the methodological framework of Arksey and O'Malley[16] and the Preferred Reporting Items for Systematic reviews and Meta-Analyses extension for Scoping Reviews (PRISMA-ScR) checklist.[17] Arksey and O'Malley (2005) describe a 6-step method that begins with identification of research question(s) and proceeds with obtaining relevant studies, developing criteria for study selection, charting the data, and summarizing and reporting the results. Research questions guide the build of the search.[16] The authors' research questions were as follows:

1. What are the experiences of AYA patients and their families in the ICU?

2. What are the experiences and perspectives of the health care professionals who care for AYA patients and their families in the ICU?
3. What are similarities and differences among the AYA stakeholder perspectives: patient, family members and healthcare professionals?

The search included adult and pediatric ICUs and all specialty ICUs with the exception of neonatal. AYAs were defined as individuals from 15 years of age to 39 years of age.[1] Although the age range for AYAs has not been defined in health care literature with consistency, AYA generally is defined based on the unique developmental needs that fit neither into the adult nor pediatric definitions. The World Health Organization (WHO) refers to "young people" as AYAs from 10 years of age to 24 years of age. The Society for Adolescent Health and Medicine uses the range of 18 years to 25 years as the definition for young adults.[4] The National Cancer Institute (NCI) defines AYAs as the group of patients between 15 years of age and 39 years of age based on the distinctive epidemiology and biology of cancers that occur in these patients. Because cancer remains one of the leading causes of death for the AYA population,[5,18] in this scoping review, the authors adopted the definition of AYA used by the NCI.

For the purposes of this review, domains of experiences were defined as psychological, spiritual, physical, emotional, financial, quality of life, well-being, communication, conflict, satisfaction, empathy, respect, and distress. To be included, a study had to examine 1 or more experience domains. Post-hospitalization studies were included if their research question was focused on the ICU experience (post-ICU recovery excluded). Only studies were included in which AYAs were a specific sample, if the mean age of the sample was between 15 years and 39 years or 1 majority of the sample was in that age range. Studies were excluded that did not report experiences, recall, or memories; reviews, case reports, editorials or opinion pieces; and dissertations. Studies were also excluded that were not written in the English language. The authors limited the search to articles published from 2010 to 2020, because AYA is a newer term in the literature.

The authors searched CINAHL, Ovid Medline, Scopus, and PsycArticles in May 2020. Search terms and complete search strategy for CINAHL are found in **Fig. 1**. In the first phase of the screening process, 3 researchers (NM, JG, and JE) independently reviewed titles and abstracts for inclusion. In the full-text phase of the process, 5 team members (NM, JG, JE, AB, an SM) independently reviewed full text articles and then discussed disagreements about inclusion until consensus (majority) was reached. Once the authors determined the articles that would be included in the scoping review, the following information was extracted from each study: design,

(adolescen* OR ((MH "Adolescent Health Services")) OR ((MH "Adolescent Medicine")) OR teen* OR ((MH "Young Adult")) OR (teenage* AND (young AND adult)) OR ((young AND adult*)) OR ((young AND person*)) OR ((young AND people)) OR AYA OR ((young AND patient*)) OR ((young AND wom*n)) OR ((young AND female*)) OR ((young AND m*n)) OR youngster* OR youth OR ((emerging AND adult)) OR ((early AND adulthood)) OR ((pre AND teen*)) OR preteen* OR ("pre adolescen*") OR preadolescen* OR ((MH "Minors (Legal)")) OR minor*) AND (((MH "Intensive Care Units+") OR "intensive care units") OR ((MH "Intensive Care Units, Neonatal")) OR ((MH "Intensive Care Units, Pediatric+")) OR ((MH "Neonatal Intensive Care Nursing")) OR ((MH "Critical Care+")) OR (intensive AND care AND unit) OR ICU) AND (("health communication") OR ((MH "Decision Making+")) OR interact* OR talk OR conversation* OR discuss* OR empathy OR ((decision AND making)) OR ("shared decision-making") OR experience OR ((MH "Professional-Patient Relations+")) OR ((MH "Anxiety+")) OR ((MH "Stress, Psychological+")) OR ((MH "Fear+")))

Fig. 1. Full search strategy from CINAHL.

sample characteristics, setting, measures, and results specific to the AYA experience in the ICU. Three members of the team (NM, JE, and JG) worked to synthesize and collate these data into an evidence table (**Table 1**). After the evidence table was complete, 3 additional team members (JP, SM, and AB) reviewed the findings to verify data extraction.

RESULTS

Of the 3627 records screened, 10 articles met all inclusion criteria (**Fig. 2**). The main reason for exclusion was lack of specificity to the AYA population.

STUDY CHARACTERISTICS
Design

Two studies[19,20] were descriptive/correlational in design. The remaining studies were qualitative, with 3 using focus groups[12,21,22] and 5 using 1-on-1 interviews[23–27] for data collection. Of these, 1 study was a qualitative evaluation of an intervention.[26]

Sample

Six studies investigated family symptoms, satisfaction, or experience,[19–24] with 1 of these studies including 9 mother/adolescent dyads.[21] The family members studied included parents, siblings, and spouses, and sample sizes ranged from 1 family unit (mother and father) to 405 family members. Three studies investigated the patient experience,[21,26,27] with sample sizes ranging from 7 to 16, including the adolescent perspective described in the mother/adolescent dyad study, referred to ptrbioudly.[21] Health care providers (nurses, physicians, allied health professionals) were interviewed in 2 studies with sample sizes of 12 to 15.[12,25]

Four studies focused on adolescents[21,23,25,26]; 2 study included younger children with adolescents[22]; 2 study included AYAs,[12] and 4 studies included samples with median/mean ages meeting inclusion criteria; however, these samples also included older adults and younger children.[19,20,24,27]

Study Setting

All studies examined some aspect of the ICU experience; 4 of the 10 studies also examined acute care experiences.[12,21,22,26] Studies were conducted in the United States[12,20,22]; Sweden[23]; United Kingdom[21,25]; Czech Republic and Slovak Republic[19]; Denmark[26]; Jordan[27]; and Turkey.[24]

Theoretic Framework

None of the studies reported a theoretical framework.

Adolescents and Young Adults Patient Experience

Two studies specifically examined adolescent experiences in the ICU[21,26] and found that their experiences were impacted by interactions with their parents and health care professionals. Adolescents want to be respected as individuals, receive information and explanations directly, and be communicated with in an age-appropriate way.[21] Adolescents reported wanting to be involved in decision making, allowed to be in control, and respected as individuals.[26] They also reported that some nurses were too busy, physicians reduced them to a diagnosis, and interacting with psychologists would associate them with the stigma of mental illness.[26] A sense of control motivated adolescents to participate/continue treatment.[26] They wanted to be known beyond their medical condition by staff[21]; get a break from their illness, treatments,

Table 1
Table of findings for scoping review

Author, Year Country	Study Aims and Framework	Study Design	Patient, Family, and Health Care Professional Perspectives and Characteristics	Setting	Measures and Analysis	Findings Related to Experience/delivery of Care for Adolescents and Young Adults
Johansson (2014)[23] Sweden	To explore the emotional responses of family members of a young adult patient in the ICU No framework (inductive approach)	Qualitative/ descriptive, case study, secondary data analysis	Family perspective Mother and father, both middle aged *Patient was a 19-year-old woman in ICU for 5 wk with pneumonia	Adult ICU	One-on-one interviews with mother and father (separately) with guiding question Hermeneutic analysis (Gadamer approach)	Six themes related to parent emotions were uncovered: 1. Feelings of uncertainty: daughter's survival and quality of life 2. Feelings of abandonment: when health care team did not allow parents by daughter's side 3. Feelings of desertion from the loved one: guilt related to inability to fulfill moral obligations to daughter 4. Feelings of being close to deathbed: processing potential death of daughter 5. Feelings of being in a no-man's land: being in disequilibrium with family roles and routine 6. Feelings of attachment: love for daughter and need to be close Other key findings: parents' extreme emotional responses—existential distress and suffering; strong need to "be with" young daughter

Author/Country	Purpose/Framework	Design	Sample	Setting	Measures/Analysis	Results
Maxim et al. (2019)[20] United States	To describe family satisfaction in a trauma and surgical ICU No framework	Descriptive	Family perspective N = 103, 75% female Median age of family member = 41 (IQR = 29–56); 45% of family sample had been in ICU in past; race and family relationship not reported but sample included both English and Spanish speaking family members. * These family members represented 88 patients: 71.6% male and 83.7% trauma injury; median age = 37.5 y; median ICU stay: 11 d	Adult ICU Trauma-surgical ICU in level i trauma center	Family satisfaction (FS-ICU 24) Demographics Mean and SD for each item and composite score	Overall high family satisfaction (M = 80.1/100; SD = 26.7) Less satisfaction surrounding items related to amount of care provided (M = 64.1; SD = 36.8), atmosphere of waiting room M = 64.8, SD = 33.3) communication between physicians and family (mean = 70.7; SD = 29.5) Open-ended comments: need for better interpreter services, accommodations for families, and more communication with physicians * Results not specific to AYAs (included older adults)
Needle et al. (2019)[12] United States	To explore the perspective of physicians in pediatric ICUs and hematopoietic stem cell transplant (HSCT) related to adolescent and young adult advance care planning and end-of-life decision making No framework (inductive approach)	Qualitative/ descriptive	HCP perspective N = 15 physicians (4 HSCT attendings; 11 pediatric ICU attendings and fellows) Mean age = 40 y (29–62 y); mean years for physician practice = 10 y (1–31 y) *The HSCT program served patients from birth to 26 y of age; focus of study was on adolescents and young adults undergoing HSCT	Pediatric ICU Large HSCT program	3 focus groups with interview guide Content analysis	Two themes uncovered: 1. The temporal context of advance care planning and decision-making: HSCT attendings: see AYA patients throughout trajectory of illness from diagnosis to death or cure. Pediatric ICU physicians: only see those with serious complications. Both groups thought conversations should occur when patients are well enough to express their values and goals as decisions

(continued on next page)

Table 1
(continued)

Author, Year Country	Study Aims and Framework	Study Design	Patient, Family, and Health Care Professional Perspectives and Characteristics	Setting	Measures and Analysis	Findings Related to Experience/delivery of Care for Adolescents and Young Adults
						about life-sustaining treatment can be different when well vs ill.

2. The limitations of pediatric advance care planning: embodied knowing (feeling and understanding) and by witnessing; the impact of clinical cascades in a new normal of aggressive, life-sustaining care; balancing AYA autonomy with capacity to make decisions; and different ways of understanding for providers, patients, and their families

Other key findings:

- Physicians felt obligated to offer life-sustaining treatment but that AYA patients may not fully understand options and consequences.
- Patients and families may learn consequences through experience of care (may not be fully informed).
- Social media plays a role in patient and

Source	Design	Purpose	Sample	Setting	Methods	Results
Robert et al. (2012)[22] United States	Qualitative, descriptive	To understand the needs and experiences of bereaved parents whose child received care at a comprehensive cancer center and determine their expectations of palliative care and how palliative care can be improved. No framework (inductive approach)	Family perspective 14 Parents of children who died a minimum of 1 y prior to participation (and child was at least 10 y of age at time of death) Mean age of parents = 51 y (SD = 6); 10 parents were white; 3 were Mexican; and 1 was Arab American *These parents represented 9 children (6 boys and 3 girls) with a mean age of 15 y (SD = 3)	Pediatric ICU and acute care	3 Focus groups using interview guide that was developed from the literature Content analysis	family decisions through communication with others in similar situations. • Physicians shared difficult emotions and felt they did not always full disclose limits of medicine because they had to be confident patient would not survive before discussing death. • Physicians base decisions on science and data; families base decisions on religious, cultural, and social constructs and how they process provided information (this can lead to conflicts regarding end of life care). Results specific to pediatric ICU: Bereaved family members reported 1. Receiving specialized attention with high support 2. Barriers to being with the child (eg, visitation rules, no chairs, no resources) 3. Feeling unclear when to return to patient from waiting room 4. Need for staff to accommodate

(continued on next page)

Table 1
(continued)

Author, Year Country	Study Aims and Framework	Study Design	Patient, Family, and Health Care Professional Perspectives and Characteristics	Setting	Measures and Analysis	Findings Related to Experience/delivery of Care for Adolescents and Young Adults
						presence of younger siblings 5. Lack of communication/information Other key findings related to family members' perspectives: • Separation from child profoundly distressing • Need for more consistent providers • Parents wanted child to have some control in end-of-life discussions; must be tailored to needs • Some providers avoided discussions about death *Not AYA specific—included younger children
Rusinova et al. (2014)[19] Czech Republic and Slovak Republic	To assess the prevalence of symptoms of anxiety and depression among family members of ICU patients; family understanding of patient condition; and identify family needs and satisfaction No framework	Descriptive/correlational	Family perspective 405 family members; median age = 41.5 y (16–87); 71.5% female; race not reported; 23% spouse; 48% parents; 15% sibling *These family members represented 293 patients with a median age = 39 y; mean ICU LOS = 13 d	17 Adult ICUs 5 Pediatric ICUs	Hospital Anxiety and Depression Scale (HADS) Critical Care Family Needs Inventory (CCFNI) Researcher developed questionnaire on information and support received Structured interview to elicit comprehension of information provided by ICU staff	The age of the patient was inversely associated with depression scores. Family members of younger patients had higher scores for depression symptoms on HADS). Family members of patients in PICUs had better comprehension of patient diagnosis

Author/Country	Design	Purpose	Setting	Sample	Methods/Analysis	Results
					Descriptive statistics, correlations, multivariate regression	than family members of patients cared for in adult ICUs (OR = 1.688, CI 1.17–2.32), $P = .008$. No differences found for anxiety and depression symptoms in family members based on the patient's care in adult vs pediatric ICU. 61.2% of family members did not understand the patient's diagnosis, features of treatment or prognosis. 27.4% wanted help from a psychologist. 17.4% received contradictory information. *Results not specific to AYAs (included older adults and children)
Seving et al. (2016)[24] Turkey	Qualitative/ descriptive	To describe the experiences of family members of patients in the ICU. No framework (inductive approach)	Adult ICU	Family perspective N = 30; 25 males and 5 females, mean age = 33 y. All were Syrian; 9 were brothers, 7 parents, 4 sons, 4 uncles, 3 spouses, and 3 of other type of relationship. *These family members represented 30 patients with a mean age of 33 (SD = 11.42)	One-on-one semistructured interviews. Demographic questionnaire. Thematic analysis	There were 6 themes about family experiences: 1. Communication-related difficulties 2. Difficulties receiving information regarding the patient's condition 3. Difficulties meeting personal needs 4. Difficulties receiving social support from other family members 5. Unmet expectations from nurses and hospital administration * Results not specific to AYAs (included older adults)

(continued on next page)

Table 1
(continued)

Author, Year Country	Study Aims and Framework	Study Design	Patient, Family, and Health Care Professional Perspectives and Characteristics	Setting	Measures and Analysis	Findings Related to Experience/delivery of Care for Adolescents and Young Adults
Villadsen et al. (2015)[26] Denmark	To describe the impact of a social-pedagogical intervention by giving adolescents the chance to talk about their experiences No framework	Qualitative/ descriptive	Patient perspective N = 7 adolescents suffering from acute or chronic critical illness Ages ranged from 14 to 20 y; LOS at time of interview ranged from 14 d to 9 mo	Adult and pediatric wards; some patients were in the ICU during hospitalization (unclear how many) *Not specific to ICUs (included acute care unit experiences)	One-on-one interviews using an interview guide Content analysis	Three themes were uncovered: 1. Recreation: adolescents appreciated physical activities offered by social educator; they valued their relationship with social educator because nurses were too busy; physicians reduced them to a diagnosis; and psychologists were associated with mental illness. 2. Structure, participation and motivation: adolescents looked forward to working with the social educator was and sessions gave them control to make decisions. This control led to motivation for their treatment and to exercise. 3. Friends and social network: It was difficult for these adolescents to keep in touch with their friends and share experiences. Working with social educator gave them something to discuss with their

	Purpose	Design	Setting	Sample	Methods/Analysis	Findings
						intervention also facilitated socialization with other hospitalized adolescents to promote normalcy. *Other key finding: adolescents talked about the importance of "getting a break" from illness, treatment, the hospital, and their overprotective parents.
Wood et al. (2018)[21] United Kingdom	To identify factors that are important to adolescents and their families during their ICU and high dependency unit (HDU) stay. No framework (inductive)	Qualitative/ descriptive	Adult and pediatric ICUs (representing 4 hospitals)	Patient and family member perspective (dyads of child and mother) There were 9 adolescents (mean age15.9 y, range of 14–19); 4 were cared for in an adult ICU and 5 in pediatric ICUs 9 mothers participated, demographics not reported 8 mother/child dyads included; 1 interview was with the mother alone.	Dyadic interviews Framework approach to analysis: familiarization, identifying thematic framework, indexing, charting, mapping and interpretation	Two factors were identified that affected the ICU experience: 1. Environment: some adolescents discussed that they were surrounded by very old people whereas others said activities on the pediatric ward were childish. 2. Staff behavior: for both adolescents and their mothers, staff behavior was central aspect of experience. Valued behaviors included: a. Inclusion: feeling involved and included in one's experience (mentioned more by pediatric ICU users) b. Providing explanations: being given information and having things explained c. Interpersonal communication: adolescents wanted staff to try to get to know them and talk to

(continued on next page)

Table 1
(continued)

Author, Year Country	Study Aims and Framework	Study Design	Patient, Family, and Health Care Professional Perspectives and Characteristics	Setting	Measures and Analysis	Findings Related to Experience/delivery of Care for Adolescents and Young Adults
						them beyond their illness. d. Tailoring communication and interaction style: adolescents described bring treated as either an adult or a child—communication more in an adult manner was preferred; they also shared they are different from both adults and from children and wanted interactions that met the needs of an adolescent. e. Respect: how staff interacted affected feeling respected—overall how care was delivered was more important than where care was received.
Wood et al. (2020)[25] United Kingdom	To explore perspectives regarding both the optimal environment (adult vs pediatric ICU) in which to care for critically ill adolescents No framework (inductive)	Qualitative/ descriptive	HCP perspectives N = 12 (6 from adult ICUs and 6 from pediatric ICUs) 6 nurses 3 consultants 3 allied health care professionals	2 adult ICUs and 2 pediatric ICUs in England	One-on-one interviews using interview guide	The main finding was, What are adolescents like? which described variable views on the adolescent by health care professionals. Two additional themes included

Median time working in ICU was 12 y (3–20 y)

1. Needs of critically ill adolescent: medical needs and the importance of delivering appropriate care, dignity and privacy, issues of consent, and minimizing the psychological impact of the ICU

2. Implications for staff: beliefs that parental presence was beneficial, lack of familiarity with the care of adolescents, and the emotional impact of caring for adolescents on health care professionals

Other key findings:

- Pediatric ICUs were more family centered, whereas adult ICUs were individual-centered care

- Duration of stay and complexity of medical needs were key considerations: adolescents who require a prolonged ICU stay should be in pediatric ICU; for short stays, adult ICUs are appropriate.

- hould consider parental presence for procedures but should be up to the adolescent

- Concerns that adolescent not fully considered in decision making

(continued on next page)

Table 1
(continued)

Author, Year Country	Study Aims and Framework	Study Design	Patient, Family, and Health Care Professional Perspectives and Characteristics	Setting	Measures and Analysis	Findings Related to Experience/delivery of Care for Adolescents and Young Adults
						• Emotional impact of caring for adolescent—death is very difficult but they also have greater chance of recovery (hopeful)
Zeilani and Seymour (2010)[27] Jordon	To describe the experiences of Muslim women in ICUs No framework (inductive approach)	Qualitative, narrative	Patient perspective 16 women included in the study from 2 different ICUs (ages 19–82 y) and of these, 8 were younger than 40 y	Adult ICU	One-on-one interviews Narrative analysis	Themes uncovered were 1. Physical suffering 2. Social suffering 3. Spiritual suffering 4. Suffering from the ICU technology *For the young adult women, social suffering was the theme most frequently described. Their children were very important to them and they thought only of their children while in the ICU. Separation from their family made them fear death and experience loneliness. They were frustrated when ICU staff did not facilitate connection with their family. *Not specific to AYAs (older adults included)

Abbreviations: IQR, interquartile range; LOS, length of stay; M, mean; PICU, pediatric ICU.

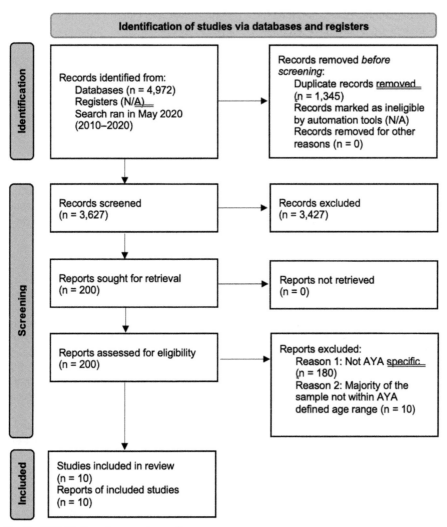

Fig. 2. PRISMA flow for search results.

and overprotective parents; and continue to be connected with their social networks and peers.[26] In Villadsen and colleagues'[26] study, adolescents who participated in a social education intervention tailored to the needs of the adolescent population with acute or chronic critical illness felt empowered to set their own goals, developed independence within the inpatient setting, and felt connected to peers. The adolescent participants developed a strong relationship with the social educator who delivered the intervention. Adolescents in the study by Wood and colleagues[21] reported that both the ICU environment and health care professionals' behaviors positively or negatively affected their experience. Adolescents felt surrounded by old people in adult ICUs, whereas in pediatric ICUs adolescents shared that activities were childish. How they were treated by health care professionals was more important to adolescents than the care setting.[21] Adolescents thought the behaviors of health care professional were positive if they made the adolescent feel included, provided information and explanations, connected them on a personal level, and tailored communication to the adolescent's needs. When these positive behaviors occurred, the adolescent felt respected. Adolescents reported being treated as either an adult or a child; while they preferred to have a more adult approach to communication, adolescents emphasized that they are different from both adults and children.[21]

One study described the experiences of women in the ICU.[27] A theme specific to the young adult (20–39 years) women in this sample was their focus on their young children. These young adults experienced extreme distress and suffering due to being separated from their children during their stay in the ICU. A participant described their important connection to their children: "I feel my children are the closest to my heart...."[27(p.170)] Their sense of purpose stemmed from their role as mother and separation from their family was intertwined with their fear of death. Mothers in this study never stopped thinking of their children, and many requested that nurses facilitate contact with their families. Nurses did not consistently respond to these requests, however, possibly not fully understanding the patients' deep need to be close to their children.

Family experience of adolescents and young adults in ICUs

Six studies described parent or family member experiences in the ICU.[19–24] There was no difference in anxiety or depression symptoms for family members related to where care was received—adult ICU versus pediatric ICU.[19] Age of the patient, however, was found inversely associated with symptoms of depression among family members (as age decreased, symptoms of depression increased).[19] In a case study in which the parents of a 19-year-old woman were interviewed about their ICU experiences, themes included a strong need to be with their daughter; uncertainty regarding her prognosis, survival, and quality of life; feeling the health care team abandoned them by not allowing them to be with their daughter; guilt that they may not be fulfilling moral obligations to her; and fluctuations in their family routines and responsibilities.[23]

Although parents recognized the high level of support and attention that their child received in the ICU setting,[22] they felt the environment posed challenges to their efforts to be at their child's bedside. Challenges included visitation rules that did not accommodate younger siblings; the ICU team's limited understanding of the needs of the entire family; lack of chairs in their child's room; extended waiting periods outside the patient room without updates and not knowing when they could return to the bedside; and lack of accommodations for family members spending prolonged periods in the hospital.[22] Although family members highly valued the information that health care professionals imparted about their child,[21] this communication was often perceived to be insufficient.[22] note, family members of patients in pediatric ICUs had better comprehension of the patient's diagnosis then those cared for in adult ICUs,[19] suggesting differences in family engagement. In the dyadic study of adolescent/mother perspectives about pediatric versus adult ICU settings, mothers, like adolescents, emphasized the importance of how providers approached interactions with their adolescent and the needs to receive information and explanations and to include parents as partners in care.[21] Mothers of adolescents surmised that a barrier to proactive palliative care was health care professionals' reluctance to broach the topic of death with a young person.[22]

Health care professionals' experience of caring for adolescents and young adults

Two studies reported the experiences of health care professionals caring for adolescents in ICUs.[12,25] Comfort in caring for adolescents and supporting their families differed among health care professionals (nurses, consultants, and allied professionals) based on their experiences caring for adolescents and knowledge about this age group.[25] These health care professionals considered the pediatric ICU better equipped to care for adolescents and their families. They reported that the decision to admit to pediatric or adult ICU should be determined by complexity of patient needs but also consider individual factors. They thought short, 1-time admissions for adolescents could be appropriate for an adult ICU, whereas chronic conditions and ongoing specialized needs were appropriate for a pediatric ICU.[25]

Health care professionals felt that caring for adolescents may have more emotional impact than caring for younger children due in part to adolescents' ability to voice concerns.[25] Involvement of adolescents in care decisions and providing explanations were considered important.[12,25] In a study of physician experiences about advance care planning with adolescents undergoing hematopoietic stem cell transplant, physicians expressed concerns about adolescents' developmental capacity to make informed decisions and also noted differences in decision-making processes among adolescent patients and their family members.[12] In both studies, health care professionals described the emotional impact of the death of an adolescent in the ICU,[12,25] especially when health care professionals are not used to caring for such young patients.[25] In the study focused on physicians caring for patients who underwent HSCT and were admitted to the ICU, physicians expressed that they need to be certain that the patient will not survive before they felt comfortable bringing up the possibility of death with an adolescent and their parents.[12]

DISCUSSION

The scoping review identified paucity of studies focused on AYA experiences in the ICU setting. The authors selected the NCI AYA definition in this review to be as broad as possible to ensure they gathered literature on both adolescent and young adult experiences. Although AYA is recognized as a distinct area of research, most studies in this scoping review focused on either adolescents or young adults. Ten studies met inclusion criteria; however, 4 of these studies[19,20,22,24] did not provide any data or analysis specific to adolescents or young adults.

A question raised in 1 of the reviewed studies was whether adolescents should be cared for in an adult ICU or a pediatric ICU.[21] In this study, adolescents reported that they cared less about the type of ICU and more about how health care professionals interacted with them and involved them as experts in their own care.[21] Beyond adolescent preferences, there is a question of whether quality of care differs for adolescents in pediatric ICUs or adult ICUs. In a large study that explored the ICU care of adolescents in the United Kingdom, adolescent mortality did not differ based on whether care was delivered in an adult ICU or a pediatric ICU.[10] Findings suggest, however, that care of adolescents in both pediatric ICU and adult ICU settings may not meet their unique needs, because they may be triaged to an adult or pediatric ICU based on their diagnoses and need for medical or surgical intervention, rather than the psychosocial factors that may influence their quality of care.[10] The question of which ICU setting is best for adolescents remains unanswered. Adolescents are a small percentage of the ICU population in both care environments,[10] posing a challenge for research. Large samples of adolescents are needed to fully examine psychosocial variables that may influence quality of care.

AYAs with complex chronic conditions have frequent interactions with the health care system and may have numerous stays in an ICU. Only 1 study in this review, however, included a sample of adolescents with chronic critical illness.[26] Adolescents with chronic conditions may have to transition from a pediatric to adult setting as they age out of pediatrics. Adolescents and their parents often feel these transitions are abrupt and perceive a lack of partnership with the health care team during this process.[28] These transitions in care represent an important opportunity for further research to elicit the needs and preferences of adolescents with chronic conditions and their families as they navigate transitions from child-focused to adult-focused care environments.

None of the reviewed studies focused solely on experiences of young adults in the ICU; however, the authors were able to cull specific data about young adult women from 1 study. An important finding from this study specific to young adult female patients was the importance of remaining connected to their children.[27] This point is illustrared in the case presented to frame the scoping review. In retrospect, the team recognized missed opportunities to facilitate Violet's connection to her children, which could have better supported her psychosocial well-being. Incorporating child life specialists who are experts in developmentally appropriate coping and psychological preparation into ICU teams could address both the needs of the young adult patient and those of any young children in their family.[29] Child life specialists have the expertise to facilitate developmentally appropriate visits with AYA patients and their children and also support the ICU team, particularly in adult ICUs, where ICU staff may be unaccustomed to involving young children in ICU visitation. Although child life specialists often are called in to assist in end-of-life situations, developing an interprofessional AYA team led by a child life specialist may be a way to address the unique needs of AYAs in the ICU setting.

This scoping review highlights that care often is not tailored to the unique needs and experiences of AYA patients.[21,26] This was emphasized in adolescents' expressed need to have health care professionals tailor their communication and interaction style to their age.[21] In this review, the uathors found that a social-pedagogical intervention that allowed adolescents to talk and clinicians to hear about the patient's personal experiences was considered helpful and motivating.[26] The authors recommend continued study of this intervention to determine if it will meet the needs of AYAs in the ICU setting.

No guidelines exist for the care of AYAs in ICUs, which is likely due to the lack of a robust evidentiary base to inform recommendations. This scoping review is a critical first step toward the development of a practice-based framework to guide ICU care for AYAs. The reviewed studies suggest that adolescents recognize their own unique needs. To ensure AYA patients and their families can fully engage as partners in care, health care professionals must address these unique needs to optimize the ICU experiences and outcomes of AYAs. Interventions cannot be developed without understanding the AYA perspective about critical care.

None of the reviewed studies describes a theoretic framework. This may be due to the inductive approach to gathering data taken by most of these studies, but it also may speak to the need for AYA-specific frameworks to guide ICU research and practice. To address the variability in ICU care for adolescents across care settings and across countries, European Society of Pediatric and Neonatal Intensive Care (ESPNIC) developed a mnemonic (the 6 Ps) to use when ICU professionals care for adolescents: privacy, permission, DVT prophylaxis, personal life, puberty, and practice issues.[30] Implementation of the 6 Ps and development of additional clinical tools are important steps toward better meeting the needs of AYAs in the ICU.

An emerging body of literature calls for the early integration of palliative care into the cancer journey of AYAs.[14,15,31,32] The authors argue that early and integrated palliative care is a critical direction for improving the care of AYAs with chronic critical illness, because exacerbations and complications of pediatric-onset chronic illnesses are reasons for ICU admissions among AYAs.[6] In a study about advance care planning for children, adolescents, and young adults with complex chronic conditions, bereaved parents valued early advance care planning, and it was associated with better quality of life.[33] There is a paucity of literature exploring the experiences of AYAs and their family members with palliative care in the ICU, including primary and specialty palliative care, serious illness communication, advance care planning, and transitions to end-of-life care. Although advance care planning before critical illness is optimal, in 1 of the studies included in this review, providers of adolescents undergoing HSCT expressed that adolescents and their families may not know what their preferences are until they experience critical illness.[12] In a study conducted in 2010, findings revealed that adolescents with leukemia or lymphoma were more likely to die in the ICU than other settings, yet end-of-life discussions were more likely to occur during the last 7 days of life.[18] Insufficient and/or delayed ICU palliative care integration continues and barriers to early and proactive palliative care consultation still are being overcome.[34,35] In 1 study the authors reviewed, parents perceived provider reluctance to discuss the possible death of their child.[22] Health care teams are tasked with balancing the developmental readiness of the adolescent for end-of-life discussions,[12] the parents' desire to protect their child from difficult conversations but also involve them in decisions about their care,[22] and health care professionals' discomfort with the potential death of a young person.[12,25] Balancing the perspectives of these three stakeholders presents unique challenges to engaging in serious illness conversations, advance care planning, and end-of-life decisions with AYAs. Specialty palliative care consultation teams have the expertise to support health care professionals, patients, and their families through the difficult emotional process of serious illness communication in the ICU.[34–36] Interprofessional palliative care teams can build the capacity of ICU teams through collaborative opportunities to learn about serious illness conversations and advance care planning for AYAs.

There were missed opportunities for primary and specialty palliative care in Violet's case, a young adult with chronic critical illness. Did this occur because the health care team had different expectations for her prognosis than they would have had for an older adult? Would advance care planning early in her illness trajectory have laid the groundwork for more palliative care involvement? Did the team fully consider this young adult's developmental stage in life and how it may influence how and who should be involved in end-of-life discussions? Research regarding the specialized palliative care needs of specific ICU populations is in its nascency and it is critical that the unique palliative care needs of AYAs are explored. Dyadic approaches to research that involve the AYA and their family member as participants in which their perspectives are elicited together and compared, such as that of Wood and colleagues,[21] could be promising given the close family relationships that may exist for AYAs. Greater insight into the experiences of AYAs in the ICU will allow palliative care to be tailored to the needs of adolescents, young adults, and their families.

This scoping review indicates critical directions for future ICU AYA research. Given the small percentage of AYAs in both adult ICU and pediatric ICU settings, future studies need to be multisite with specific samples of AYA ICU patients and their families. The authors propose the following research questions:

1. Do critically ill AYA patients have a more severe psychological symptom burden compared with older critically ill patients?
2. Are AYA family members more likely to support life-sustaining interventions, such as mechanical ventilation, dialysis, vasopressor support, and cardiopulmonary resuscitation for critically ill AYA patients, compared with older critically ill adults?
3. What is the frequency of identifying a surrogate decision maker (SDM) among critically ill AYA patients compared with older critically ill adults? Who are the SDMs for critically ill AYAs?

4. What are the unique communication/interpersonal dynamics of critically ill AYA patients and their families and health care providers, compared with non-AYA patients?
5. What are the perspectives of health care professionals in pediatric ICUs and adult ICUs regarding caring for the chronically critically ill AYA population?
6. Could a Delphi approach with AYA patients, families, and health care professionals be used to further understand the unique needs of this distinct ICU population and begin to lay the foundation for the development of practice guidelines for AYA ICU care?
7. In what ways do the perspectives of AYA patients and their family members about advance care planning change in the context of critical illness?

LIMITATIONS OF THIS REVIEW

This review was limited to case studies and primary research in the English language; therefore, findings may not represent all languages/cultures. Only 10 studies met inclusion criteria due to a paucity of literature in this area and/or limitations of the search strategy. Although AYAs may be included in adult ICU or pediatric ICU research, samples of ICU patients tend to be heterogenous with only a small percentage of AYA patients; thus, it is difficult to distinguish differences among the experiences of children, adolescents, young adults, and adults. Becuase professional bodies define the age range of AYA differently, researchers may focus on differing age ranges when studying adolescents, young adults, or AYAs, which makes comparison of findings in the AYA literature more challenging. The authors applied the NCI definition of the AYA age range for article inclusion; thus, the scoping review findings might be different if another definition of AYA had been applied.

SUMMARY

In conclusion, this scoping review underscores the limited literature specific to adolescents, particularly to young adults in the ICU setting. The authors' analysis of the perspectives of patients, family members, and health care professionals indicates that the unique developmental needs of adolescents, and likely young adults, may not be adequately met. Further insights are needed to seize opportunities to tailor ICU care to the developmental stage of the AYA population and improve family-centered care. Without further exploratory research, the unique needs of AYAs and their families will remain poorly understood. Additionally, the scoping review suggests that strengthening ICU professionals' serious illness communication skills may improve the experience of AYAs and their families in the ICU and may decrease the distress of the health care professionals caring for this population.

CLINICS CARE POINTS

- From the adolescent and parent perspective, it may be less important where an adolescent is cared for (pediatric ICU vs adult ICU) and may be more important that an adolescent is treated as a unique individual.
- AYA patients and their family members need to be fully engaged in care, and the health care team needs to provide family-centered support.
- ICU teams need access to AYA experts, such as child life specialists and palliative care specialists, to inform and guide their serious illness conversations with AYAs and their family members.

• Evidence is needed to develop practice guidelines for AYA care in both adult ICU and pediatric ICU settings.

DISCLOSURE

This project was funded by an internal grant from the University of Wisconsin-Milwaukee – The Collaborative Research Team Development Award (AAG7969).

REFERENCES

1. National Cancer Institute. Adolescents and Young Adults (AYAs) with cancer - National Cancer Institute. Published May 15, 2015. Available at: https://www.cancer.gov/types/aya. [Accessed 9 July 2021].
2. World Health Organization. Adolescence: a period needing special attention - recognizing-adolescence. Published 2021. Available at: https://apps.who.int/adolescent/second-decade/section2/page1/recognizing-adolescence.html. [Accessed 9 July 2021].
3. Berger K. The developing person through the life span. 11th edition. Macmillan Learning for Instructors. Macmillan Learning; 2020. Available at: https://www.macmillanlearning.com/college/us/product/The-Developing-Person-Through-the-Life-Span/p/1319191754. [Accessed 29 July 2021].
4. Society for Adolescent Health and Medicine. Young adult health and well-being: a position statement of the society for adolescent health and medicine. J Adolesc Health 2017;60(6):758–9.
5. Centers for Disease Control and Prevention. Injuries and violence are leading causes of death. Published March 9, 2021. Available at: https://www.cdc.gov/injury/wisqars/animated-leading-causes.html. [Accessed 8 July 2021].
6. West JC, Bush K, Trayhan M, et al. Young adults in the intensive care unit: a unique high-risk population. In: A36. Hot topics in critical care medicine. American Thoracic Society International Conference Abstracts. American Thoracic Society; 2018. p. A1468. https://doi.org/10.1164/ajrccm-conference.2018.197.1_MeetingAbstracts.A1468.
7. Vizient. CDB | healthcare analytics platform for clinical benchmarking. Published 2021. Available at: https://www.vizientinc.com/our-solutions/clinical-solutions/clinical-data-base. [Accessed 29 July 2021].
8. Bohula EA, Katz JN, van Diepen S, et al. Demographics, care patterns, and outcomes of patients admitted to cardiac intensive care units: the Critical Care Cardiology Trials Network Prospective North American Multicenter Registry of Cardiac Critical Illness. JAMA Cardiol 2019;4(9):928.
9. Society of Critical Care Medicine. SCCM | critical care statistics. Society of Critical Care Medicine (SCCM); 2021. Available at: https://sccm.org/Communications/Critical-Care-Statistics. [Accessed 8 July 2021].
10. Wood D, Goodwin S, Pappachan J, et al. Characteristics of adolescents requiring intensive care in the United Kingdom: a retrospective cohort study. J Intensive Care Soc 2018;19(3):209–13.
11. Mack JW, Chen K, Boscoe FP, et al. High intensity of end-of-life care among adolescent and young adult cancer patients in the New York State Medicaid Program. Med Care 2015;53(12):1018–26.
12. Needle JS, Peden-McAlpine C, Liaschenko J. Physicians' perspectives on adolescent and young adult advance care planning. Fallacy Informed Decis Making 2019;30(2):12.

13. Lima L, Gonçalves S, Pinto C. Sudden death in paediatrics as a traumatic experience for critical care nurses: sudden death in paediatrics. Nurs Crit Care 2018; 23(1):42–7.
14. Pinkerton R, Donovan L, Herbert A. Palliative care in adolescents and young adults with cancer—why do adolescents need special attention? Cancer J 2018;24(6):336–41.
15. Upshaw NC, Roche A, Gleditsch K, et al. Palliative care considerations and practices for adolescents and young adults with cancer. Pediatr Blood Cancer 2021; 68(1):e28781.
16. Arksey H, O'Malley L. Scoping studies: towards a methodological framework. Int J Social Res Methodol 2005;8(1):19–32.
17. Tricco AC, Lillie E, Zarin W, et al. PRISMA extension for scoping reviews (PRISMA-ScR): checklist and explanation. Ann Intern Med 2018;169(7):467.
18. Bell CJ, Skiles J, Pradhan K, et al. End-of-life experiences in adolescents dying with cancer. Support Care Cancer 2010;18(7):827–35.
19. Rusinova K, Kukal J, Simek J, et al. Limited family members/staff communication in intensive care units in the Czech and Slovak Republics considerably increases anxiety in patients   relatives – the DEPRESS study. BMC Psychiatry 2014; 14(1):21.
20. Maxim T, Alvarez A, Hojberg Y, et al. Family satisfaction in the trauma and surgical intensive care unit: another important quality measure. Trauma Surg Acute Care Open 2019;4(1):e000302.
21. Wood D, Geoghegan S, Ramnarayan P, et al. Eliciting the experiences of the adolescent-parent dyad following critical care admission: a pilot study. Eur J Pediatr 2018;177(5):747–52.
22. Robert R, Zhukovsky DS, Mauricio R, et al. Bereaved parents' perspectives on pediatric palliative care. J Soc Work End Life Palliat Care 2012;8(4):316–38.
23. Johansson I. Emotional responses of family members of a critically ill patient: a hermeneutic analysis. Int J Emerg Ment Health 2014;16(1):213–6.
24. Sevinç S, Ajghif M, Uzun Ö, et al. Expectations of relatives of Syrian patients in intensive care units in a state hospital in Turkey. J Clin Nurs 2016;25(15–16): 2232–41.
25. Wood D, Geoghegan S, Ramnarayan P, et al. Where should critically ill adolescents receive care? A qualitative interview-based study of perspectives of staff working in adult and pediatric intensive care units. J Intensive Care Med 2020; 35(11):1271–7.
26. Villadsen KW, Blix C, Boisen KA. More than a break: the impact of a social-pedagogical intervention during young persons' long-term hospital admission – a qualitative study. Int J Adolesc Med Health 2015;27(1):19–24.
27. Zeilani R, Seymour JE. Muslim women's experiences of suffering in Jordanian intensive care units: a narrative study. Intensive Crit Care Nurs 2010;26(3): 175–84.
28. Coyne I, Sheehan A, Heery E, et al. Healthcare transition for adolescents and young adults with long-term conditions: qualitative study of patients, parents and healthcare professionals' experiences. J Clin Nurs 2019;28(21–22):4062–76.
29. Crider J, Pate MFD. Helping children say goodbye to loved ones in adult and pediatric intensive care units: certified child life specialist—critical care nurse partnership. AACN Adv Crit Care 2011;22(2):109–12.
30. Tuckwell R, Wood D, Mansfield-Sturgess S, et al. A European Society of Paediatric and Neonatal Intensive Care (ESPNIC) survey of European critical care management of young people. Eur J Pediatr 2017;176(2):155–61.

31. Avery J, Geist A, D'Agostino NM, et al. "It's more difficult...": clinicians' experience providing palliative care to adolescents and young adults diagnosed with advanced cancer. JCO Oncol Pract 2020;16(1):e100–8.

32. Barr RD, Ferrari A, Ries L, et al. Cancer in adolescents and young adults: a narrative review of the current status and a view of the future. JAMA Pediatr 2016; 170(5):495.

33. DeCourcey DD, Silverman M, Oladunjoye A, et al. Advance care planning and parent-reported end-of-life outcomes in children, adolescents, and young adults with complex chronic conditions*. Crit Care Med 2019;47(1):101–8.

34. Aulisio MP, Chaitin E, Arnold RM. Ethics and palliative care consultation in the intensive care unit. Crit Care Clin 2004;20(3):505–23.

35. McAndrew N, Guttormson J, Marks S, et al. ICU nurse: could we call a palliative care consult? ICU provider: it's too early. Palliative care integration in the ICU: the struggle to translate evidence into practice. Dimens Crit Care Nurs 2021;40(1): 51–8. https://doi.org/10.1097/DCC.0000000000000451.

36. Hartjes TM. Making the case for palliative care in critical care. Crit Care Nurs Clin North Am 2015;27(3):289–95.

Hearing their Voice
Advance Care Planning for the Homeless

Delia M. Cortez, MSW, LCSW, LICSW, APHSW-C[a],[1],
Jeannette Meyer, MSN, RN, CCRN-K, CCNS, PCCN-K, ACHPN[b],*

KEYWORDS

- Homeless • People experiencing homelessness • Advance directive
- Advance care planning • Dying • End of life

KEY POINTS

- Homeless individuals are at high risk of dying in inpatient settings.
- Homeless individuals are seldom engaged in Advance Care Planning.
- Homeless individuals welcome the opportunity to complete an advance directive.
- Trust with homeless individuals is more easily established in a familiar setting.

INTRODUCTION: HOMELESSNESS AND THE IMPACT ON CRITICAL CARE

An unidentified man is found in cardiac arrest behind a local store. Bystander CPR is initiated and an ambulance is called to transport the man to the hospital. When the ambulance arrives, the Emergency Medical Technicians (EMTs) determine he is in ventricular fibrillation and he is defibrillated with 200 J, and given epinephrine without effect, then intubated. Advance Cardiac Life Support (ACLS) continues as he is transported to an area Academic Medical Center.

Upon arrival, although ACLS continues, a social worker searches through the man's clothing. He has been found to be wearing 2 layers of shirts and pants and has a small amount of money in his inside pocket along with some unidentified medications and a bottle holding an unidentified liquid that smells strongly of alcohol. No identification is found and he had no other belongings with him. His shoes are in tatters.

As the team is preparing to stop the code, return of spontaneous circulations (ROSC) is obtained. The man, now "John Doe 230," is transported to critical care, placed on a hypothermia protocol with amiodarone and levophed infusions, sedated with propofol, and provided with a low-dose fentanyl infusion for pain control. He

[a] Licensed Clinical Social Worker for Palliative Care at UCLA Health, Los Angeles, CA, USA;
[b] Clinical Nurse Specialist for Palliative Care at UCLA Health, Los Angeles, CA, USA
[1] Present address: 1328 16th Street, 2nd Floor, (Mail Code 703646), Santa Monica, CA 90404.
* Corresponding author. 1328 16th Street. 2nd Floor, (Mail Code 703646), Santa Monica, CA 90404.
E-mail address: jmeyer@mednet.ucla.edu

appears not to have bathed or shaved in some time and his oral hygiene is poor. The pills are identified as oxycodone.

As days progress, with the assistance of local police and homeless rescue and resource centers in the area and the tireless work of social workers, the unfortunate man gradually obtains an identity. He is Jacob Ryan, a 55-year-old homeless man who has been in the area for little more than a year. Other than a small group of friends at a local park with whom he uses drinks, he keeps to himself. He has never mentioned family.

Tragically, his prognosis is extremely poor; a myocardial infarction is found to have likely caused the cardiac arrest, possibly precipitated by cocaine use. Even if Jacob survives, his anoxic brain injury will leave him in a dependent state with a tracheostomy and feeding tube, likely ventilator dependent. The social workers are able to locate one sibling, but he wants nothing to do with his brother or any decisions that need to be made.

By now more than a week has passed; Jacob remains extremely unstable, with secondary sepsis developing due to pneumonia. Pain control is difficult because of a labile blood pressure that drops when medication is given. The critical care team appeals to the hospital ethicist; who reviews the case. The team is asking for permission to withdraw life-prolonging treatment and provide comfort care. An ethics committee is convened, and they support the critical care team recommendation. Jacob is made to Unilateral Do Not Resuscitate (No Compressions or Defibrillation), but hospital policy requires a 10-day wait while additional effort is made to locate family members. In that interim, another critical care attending assumes care who is reluctant to withdraw because of his own beliefs. The frustrated bedside nurses and other caregivers continue to support Jacob, who is now poorly responsive even without sedation.

Ultimately Jacob is transferred to a skilled nursing facility. He continues to return to the hospital at intervals with bouts of sepsis, urinary tract infections, and pneumonia. No additional family willing to make decisions for him is ever found.

This tragic scenario takes place on the streets and in hospital settings throughout the country. Patients like Jacob, trapped in a medical maelstrom without an end, find themselves with a quality of life that they likely would never have wanted. But imagine now if Jacob had met volunteers from the *Hearing their Voice* volunteer team and been given an opportunity to make his wishes known. The ending of this story might have been very different for all involved.

In the bottom of Jacob's pocket, the social workers find a small green piece of paper that indicates that Jacob has completed an advance directive. He lists no one to be called, but checks off 3 local rescues where he receives assistance. The social workers are able to obtain a copy of the directive from the first of these; it states clearly in rather awkward writing that Jacob values his independence and would not want life-prolonging treatment and resuscitation if he could not make his own decisions. He does not want his family called. He would want to be made comfortable at the end of his life. He also mentions that he enjoys rock music. The directive has the 2 necessary witness signatures to be legal.

An ethics committee meeting is in unanimous agreement that Jacob's directive must be honored. Life-prolonging treatment is withdrawn and Jacob is placed on comfort care. He dies peacefully a few hours later with rock music playing in his room.

ADVANCE CARE PLANNING OVERVIEW

Advance care planning (ACP) is defined as "extending a person's autonomy by allowing individuals, particularly those with progressive illness, to reflect on and articulate their preferences for medical care in advance of medical crises that might impede their ability to speak for themselves. Through the mechanisms of open communication and the explicit documentation of preferences, ACP can help patients and families have greater control over how and where they engage with the health care system."[1] ACP involves discussions that are ideally reflected in an Advance Health Care Directive (AHCD), which is a form that allows a person to appoint a power of attorney for health care (health care agent) and write health care instructions to guide your health care agent and health care providers. The AHCD is for health care, not financial or fiduciary power of attorney. This is often not understood and a financial directive requires a different form.[2]

Although ACP is promoted as being available for all, there are identified barriers for both domiciled and people experiencing homelessness (PEH) alike. For instance, despite having regular primary care visits, less than 5% of patients will be engaged in an ACP discussion by their provider[3]. For PEH additional barriers impacting their engaging in ACP include years of homelessness, increased social isolation, limited opportunities for discussion with friends/family, obtaining food and shelter, and time constraints[3].

One of the interventions that have been successful with this population has been *outreach*. Webster's dictionary[4] defines this as the "act of reaching out; the extending of services or assistance beyond current or usual limits an outreach program also; the extent of such services or assistance." Outreach has been found to increase success as defined by engaging in related discussion and AHCD completion.[5]

PREVALENCE AND INCIDENCE: HOW COMMON IS HOMELESSNESS?

Homelessness is described as a person who lacks a fixed, regular, and adequate nighttime residence.[6] Within this definition, there are two groups identified as unsheltered and sheltered homeless. Unsheltered refers to people whose primary nighttime location is a public or private place not designated for, or ordinarily used as, a regular sleeping accommodation for people (eg, the streets, vehicles, or parks). Sheltered refers to people who are staying in emergency shelters, transitional housing programs, or safe havens.[6]

The 2020 Annual Homeless Assessment Report (AHAR) to Congress found more than half of all PEH in the United States were primarily in 4 states: California (28% or 161,548 people); New York (16% or 91,271 people); Florida (5% or 27,487 people); and Texas (5% or 27,229). California accounted for more than half of all unsheltered people in the country (51% or 113,660 people), a 10,270 increase between 2019 and 2020. This is nearly 9 times the number of unsheltered people in the state with the next highest number, Texas. States in the west reported the highest percentages of all PEH in unsheltered locations. In California, 70% of PEH did so outdoors. The 2020 single night count or point in time count in Los Angeles County, which will be the area focus of this article, found the majority of those experiencing homeless were individuals and unsheltered.[6]

For the purpose of this article, the focus will be Service Planning Area 5 (SPA), a specific geographic region within Los Angeles County.[7] This area includes Westside communities Beverly Hills, Brentwood, Culver City, Malibu, Pacific Palisades, Playa del Rey, Santa Monica, and Venice. UCLA Santa Monica Medical Center, an academic medical center with 281 inpatient beds with an average length of stay of 5 days.[8] In 2019, there were approximately 90,401 total residents in Santa Monica, CA.[9] The January 2020 homeless count found 907 PEH in Santa Monica. About 600 were unsheltered and 300 were living in shelters or institutions. The number of people counted on the beach and in downtown Santa Monica decreased by 14% in 2020 following a 19% decrease the previous year. The city's homeless population grew by 3% in 2019 and 4% in 2018 after jumping 26% in 2017.

BACKGROUND: A DESTINATION FOR HOMELESSNESS

On any given day or night, UCLA Santa Monica Medical Center, an academic medical center, treats 300 PEH a month in our emergency room. It is located in SPA 5 (service planning areas are a way in which Homeless Outreach Organizations can monitor and plan their work). SPA 5 includes Beverly Hills, Brentwood, Culver City, Malibu, Pacific Palisades, Playa del Rey, Santa Monica, and Venice.[10] These communities reflect what occurs on a larger scale, addressing the barriers to engaging marginalized populations in ACP. Experiencing chronic homelessness has been found to lead to shortened life expectancy,[11] increase in medical needs, and barriers to health care,[10] which are of particular interest for those of us in health care. Despite these factors, homeless persons are aging, requiring more attention to palliative care, hospice, end-of-life care culminating in ACP.[11]

CONSIDERATIONS: A HIGH-RISK POPULATION

Homelessness itself is a risk factor for a critical care placement.[12] PEH, especially those who are older, have many of the same chronic conditions that the domiciled have; conditions such as diabetes, hypertension, heart failure, renal failure, and liver failure. Compounding these chronic conditions may be additional extenuating factors such as mental illness and substance abuse. PEH face multiple challenges in pursuing appropriate health care for chronic conditions.[13] These challenges, as shared by the PEH, that we have interviewed in the course of our project and confirmed by literature,[13] include: difficulty obtaining a primary physician and getting to appointments; challenges with obtaining nutritious and balanced meals; challenges with obtaining prescriptions and supplies and storing these in a safe and environmentally appropriate place; harsh living conditions, including heat and cold, for PEH who are unable or unwilling to use shelters. These many pre-existing health care conditions and the challenges PEH face place them at high risk for exacerbations, which may lead to their admission to critical care. And for many PEH, there is a risk of violence inherent in their unprotected surroundings; some of those we have spoken with in the course of our project refuse to go to shelters because they have experienced assault and rape there as well. The Downtown Women's Center in Los Angeles County interviewed its clients in 2019 and learned that 60% of women experiencing homelessness had experienced violence and 23% reported feeling unsafe in shelters.[14]

DISCUSSION: WHO WE ARE

The Palliative Care Licensed Clinical Social Worker (LCSW) and Clinical Nurse Specialist (CNS) at an urban academic medical center have had training in ACP and it was a regular part of our practice. We noted in the scope of our work that our homeless patients were not being offered the opportunity to express their values and desires related to end-of-life care, which is ACP. This realization was confirmed by obtaining feedback from UCLA's hospital-based homelessness discussion group, homeless advocates' panel which the palliative care team hosted.

The general perception was that PEH would indeed be interested in ACP, including AHCD completion, naming a decision maker, and specifying their health care instructions.[15] From this point, our project expanded its multidisciplinary approach to ensure our primary goal was to extend and normalize ACP to PEH as had been done with other groups.

In 2014, the workgroup known as the UCLA SM Social Action Workgroup obtained a grant through the Coalition of Compassionate Care of California that would support the workgroup members to train others on ACP and delivery of the curriculum and education we envisioned developing and providing. We were then able to develop a program that would come to have 3 main branches: (1) direct ACP discussions with those experiencing homelessness, (2) ACP training for community agencies that service those experiencing homelessness, and (3) Hospice Under The Bridge which would take end-of-life care directly to the streets.

Direct ACP

Initially, we collectively decided to start with providing ACP direct education with PEH. We began within our own institution, strategically joining with medical units that had higher numbers of patients experiencing homelessness. For PEH, routine primary care is not an option for various reasons, resulting in increased emergency department (ED) room visits and acute hospitalizations.[16] Knowing this, we focused on challenging the cycle of the ED visit-admission-discharge cycle by attempting to interrupt it. We developed a process in which they would alert us to a patient admission that met the following criteria: (1) Homelessness, which was defined as "lacking a fixed or adequate nighttime residence". (2) Intact capacity, no cognitive barriers to making own decisions, (3) not under the influence of a chemical substance, (4) not conserved or other legal guardianship in place, (5) 18 years of age and older or an emancipated minor, (6) a psychiatric diagnosis and language were not barriers to potential engagement, this would, however, require further assessment and resources by the ACP providers. We soon found that inpatient outreach was not successful because most did not meet the established criteria as well as time limitations. This made us realize that the location of engaging PEH would be important to the success of ACP engagement.

We continued our direct engagement with PEH at a local food bank in SPA 5, led by the Palliative Care Clinical Nurse Specialist and volunteers, which proved to be successful. We have learned that people experiencing homeless do want to be engaged in ACP and have specific needs they want to be heard and documented, which is contrary to previous beliefs.[5] This weekend only foodbank is a dynamic place that allows for people experiencing homeless to congregate over a meal, pick up donated clothing and toiletries, and connect with one another. We were able to add resource connection and ACP to the existing services. Being in a place that "belonged" to the PEH allowed us to develop rapport and trust with the clients that led to meaningful ACP education, exploration, and discussions. The efforts of the foodbank outreach team are partially reflected in the number of goals of care conversations held, which are approximately 700 people and 500 AHCD provided.

The AHCD used for this project is *Prepare for Your Care's California Healthcare Directive*.[16] At the beginning of this project, 25 local community representatives were asked to review 3 AHCDs to determine which would be the most appropriate for this project and its recipients. The AHCDs included the California Hospital Association's AHCD,[17] UCLA's AHCD,[18] and Prepare for Your Care's California Health Care Directive. Owing to the sixth-grade language used, ease of use, accessibility, and bilingual versions available, the California Health Care Directive was selected. It should be noted patients are educated there are various versions of an AHCD and provided such if requested to do so. Thus far, it has been well received by patients and volunteers alike.

Collaboration Through Education

As our outreach efforts continued, we realized educating the community agency staff would be a significant part of sustaining the ACP project. Anecdotally, it was known the relationship between community CM and client was special in the sense that it held trust which allowed for a vulnerable space, a needed ingredient in ACP. We knew, and hoped, our patients would take the ACP education we had introduced them to their community CM, which we actually hoped they would do to continue the discussion. Therefore, it was important to align with them through education. During our educational presentations, we identified there was a lack of ACP knowledge and priority among the staff in the local community agencies. They did not have the language for proper follow-up nor initiate an ACP discussion. Unfortunately, this is a common finding because of other competing factors taking priority. In addition, both housed and not housed clients report feeling uncomfortable initiating an ACP conversation with a provider or do not know how to continue an ACP discussion, therefore developing the knowledge among the community agencies was imperative.[11] However, through tailored education and training the content for this client population, it is now a part of their assessment, especially for those who are high hospital utilizers. Studies have demonstrated that providing assistance with AHCD completion lead to higher completion rates as compared for self-initiated AHCDs.[19]

Placement: Hospice Under the Bridge

As we progressed in our project, common trends began to appear among our PEH who were discussing and completing directives. They wanted to die in comfort, be treated with dignity, and have their friends able to visit them. Unfortunately, these options often contrasted with the reality of what PEH experienced in our area. In Los Angeles County in 2020, 1383 PEH died; of those, most died in settings such as tents, under freeways, in alleys, or in their cars.[20] A total of 293 PEH died in hospital settings; although the study we cite mentions that some had hospice care, they do not differentiate those who died with hospice support or those who died in critical care settings.[20]

Some PEH are admitted to long-term care facilities when they are unable to care for themselves; however, in our area, even before the COVID-19 outbreak that restricted visitation to so many facilities, some of the PEH we spoke to mentioned challenges and resistance if they attempted to visit their friends who were in facilities. (Note: this is anecdotal data only.)

The CNS launched "Hospice Under the Bridge"; a networking coalition of like-minded health care and community members who worked together to seek solutions to the issue of allowing dying PEH a place where they could be comfortable and receive hospice support in their final days. Key players in this enterprise included 3 hospices who felt drawn to the care of the homeless; one of these hospices also developed a specialty in caring PEH who wanted to remain in their setting of choice for as long as possible.

A team of our collaborators were able to secure a grant and create a training and care program for dying PEH in 3 of the Respite Care Centers across Los Angeles called Brilliant Corners. The 3 hospices who were part of Hospice Under the Bridge were able to partner with them to offer education and end-of-life care to their employees and provide the needed hospice care. In addition, the CNS provided education on AHCDs for these respite organizations, Los Angeles Homeless Services Authority (LAHSA) team members, and other community agencies to assist in the project. Although still in its infancy, this project is showing great promise.

SUMMARY

PEH are seldom offered the opportunity to complete advance directives and designate decision makers. During a catastrophic illness, health care providers are left to do aggressive, life-prolonging treatments that the patient may not want while seeking decision makers who may not be familiar with the patient or what their wishes would be. If given an opportunity and approached in a setting where they feel secure, PEH are receptive to learning about Advance Care Planning and exploring advance directives. They would also prefer to die in a comfortable setting with as much autonomy as possible, though many communities lack the resources to care for dying homeless patients in a setting they would prefer.

Further research, outreach, and support systems are needed to provide homeless patients with the decision-making opportunities and end-of-life care that they deserve.

PEARLS AND PITFALLS
Pearls

- If given the opportunity, PEH often welcome the chance to complete an Advance Health Care Directive.
- Trust is an absolute necessity and may take time to establish.
- Discussing ACP and AHCDs in a setting that PEH are familiar with, such as a local food bank, shelter, or outreach center, is more effective than approaching the topic during an inpatient stay.
- If the PEH does not have a decision maker, recording their medical treatment and quality of life preferences is extremely important.
- An AHCD written at a lower literacy level (eg, fifth grade level) is preferred for this population.
- Outreach, including follow-up, increases the success rate in PEH engaging in ACP discussions and AHCD completion.
- Like many others, PEH value comfort and dignity at end of life. They also prefer a setting that honors their autonomy

Pitfalls

- Although many PEH would want comfort and dignity at end of life, there are few resources in many communities that can meet the needs of this population.
- If there are health care myths or reasons for distrust, these need to be alleviated and debunked if an outreach project is to succeed. For example, there was an initial misconception among the PEH our team worked with that the AHCD would allow our hospital system to "steal their organs."
- Depending on the resources available in your area, having the AHCD available and easily accessible to area health care systems may be challenging. Before initiating an outreach, network with local outreach resources, including city and county, and determine if there are ways that the AHCD can be stored on their databases.
- Hard copies of the AHCD are easily lost. On the advice of the PEH that we served, our team created a small green distinctive-looking piece of paper that would list the individual's name, their decision maker or emergency contact (if any), if they have an AHCD and locations where the AHCD is on file. Even if the client is robbed or separated from their belongings, this small piece of paper could be found in their pocket.

- An AHCD will likely not prevent an initial resuscitation effort, but locating it may allow the client's medical preferences to be followed and their decision maker to be located.

ACKNOWLEDGEMENTS

Coalition for Compassionate Care of California which provided our initial funding.

DISCLOSURE

The authors have nothing to disclose.

ADDITIONAL RESOURCES

Coalition for Compassionate Care of California. Available at: https://coalitionccc.org/common/Uploaded%20files/PDFs/snapshot_advance_care_planning.pd. Accessed July 22, 2021.

ACP forms. Available at: https://www.uclahealth.org/advance-care-planning/advance-directive-forms. Accessed July 22, 2021.

Sudore RL, Cuervo IA, Tieu L, et al. Advance care planning for older homeless-experienced adults: results from the health outcomes of people experiencing homelessness in older middle age study. J Am Geriatr Soc 2018;66(6):1068–74.

"Outreach." Merriam-Webster.com. 2021. Available at: https://www.merriam-webster.com. Accessed July 22, 2021.

Song J, Ratner ER, Wall MM, et al. Effect of an End-of-Life Planning Intervention on the completion of advance directives in homeless persons: a randomized trial. Ann Intern Med 2010;153(2):76–84.

Henry M, De Sousa T, Roddey C, et al. The annual homeless assessment report to congress (2020). SSRN Electron J 2021;1–102. https://doi.org/10.2139/ssrn.1680873. Available at: https://www.huduser.gov/portal/sites/default/files/pdf/2020-AHAR-Part-1.pdf.

Community and Field services Division. Available at: http://publichealth.lacounty.gov/chs/SPAMain/ServicePlanningAreas.htm#:~:text=A%20Service%20Planning%20Area%2C%20or,divided%20into%208%20geographic%20areas. Accessed July 22, 2021.

By the numbers. Available at: https://www.uclahealth.org/santa-monica/by-the-numbers. Accessed July 22, 2021.

U.S. Census Bureau QuickFacts: Santa Monica city, California; United States. (n.d.). Census Bureau QuickFacts. Available at: https://www.census.gov/quickfacts/fact/table/santamonicacitycalifornia,US/PST04521. Accessed July 22, 2021.

Hwang SW, Tolomiczenko G, Kouyoumdjian FG, et al. Interventions to improve the health of the homeless: a systematic review. Am J Prev Med 2005;29(4):311–9.

Song J, Wall MM, Ratner ER, et al. Engaging homeless persons in end of life preparations. J Gen Intern Med 2008;23(12):2031–6 [quiz: 2037–45].

Norris WM, Nielsen EL, Engelberg RA, et al. Treatment preferences for resuscitation and critical care among homeless persons. Chest 2005;127(6):2180–7.

Death on the street: homeless population is getting older and sicker. Available at: https://www.salon.com/2016/04/14/death_on_the_street_americas_homeless_population_is_growing_older_and_sicker_partner/. Accessed July 28. 2021.

Violence against Women: Domestic violence and homelessness. Available at: https://downtownwomenscenter.org/violence-against-women/. Accessed July 28, 2021.

Advance care planning: Health Care Directives. Available at: https://www.nia.nih.gov/health/advance-care-planning-health-care-directives. Accessed July 22, 2021.

Prepare for your care California Advance Healthcare Directive. Available at: https://prepareforyourcare.org/welcome. Accessed July 22, 2021.

Advance Health Care Directive. Available at: https://www.ccsombudsman.org/wp-content/uploads/2018/02/ahcd.pdf. Accessed July 22, 2021.

UCLA Health Advance Healthcare Directive. Available at: https://www.uclahealth.org/Workfiles/site/AdvanceDirective_English.pdf. Accessed July 22, 2021.

Tarzian AJ, Neal MT, O'Neil JA. Attitudes, experiences, and beliefs affecting end-of-life decision-making among homeless individuals. J Palliat Med 2005;8(1):36–48.

Ward, Ethan. February 10, 2021. Available at: https://xtown.la/2021/02/10/homeless-deaths-los-angeles/. Accessed July 28, 2021.

Palliative Care and Population Management Compassionate Extubation of the ICU Patient and the Use of the Respiratory Distress Observation Scale

Karin Cooney-Newton, MSN, RN, APRN, ACCNS-AG, CCRN[a],*,
Erin C. Hare, MSN, RN, CCRN[b]

KEYWORDS

- End-of-Life • Compassionate extubation • Ventilator withdrawal
- Terminal ventilator wean • RDOS • Respiratory distress observation scale

KEY POINTS

- Compassionate extubation (CE) is new terminology for "terminal wean" or "ventilator withdrawal" or "terminal extubation."
- Guidelines and algorithms assist staff in maintaining a coordinated, structured process at end of life (EOL), and these help create a less stressful environment for the patient, their families, and health care staff.
- The Respiratory Distress Observation Scale (RDOS) is an evidence-based, objective tool that helps to validate the need for medication titration for comfort during CE and EOL care.
- Using RDOS and CE guidelines, the critical care nurse and the respiratory therapist work together decreasing ventilator support incrementally while maintaining the RDOS goal of less than 4 to prevent and minimize patient distress.

INTRODUCTION

End-of-life (EOL) patient care can be an extremely stressful experience for not only the patients, but also their families and the health care team. When training to become a critical care nurse, the focus is largely on helping patients survive acute episodes and assisting in restoring their health. Unfortunately, not all patients are able to fully recover, or return to their desired quality of life. Studies show that 22% of all deaths

---

[a] Bayhealth Medical Center, 640 S State Street, Mail code: 1207, Dover, DE 19901, USA; [b] MICU, ChristianaCare Hospital, 4755 Ogletown-Stanton Road, Newark, DE 19718, USA
* Corresponding author.
E-mail address: Karin_cooney-newton@bayhealth.org

Crit Care Nurs Clin N Am 34 (2022) 67–78
https://doi.org/10.1016/j.cnc.2021.11.004
0899-5885/22/© 2021 Elsevier Inc. All rights reserved.

in the United States (before the COVID-19 pandemic) occur in or after admission to an intensive care unit (ICU).[1] The health care team must transition these patients from restorative care to palliative care. It is considered one of the most difficult and important aspects of nursing practice in the ICU setting.[1]

BACKGROUND

Compassionate extubation (CE) is termination of mechanical ventilation and withdrawal of an artificial airway to avoid prolonged suffering at end of life (EOL). The CE experience can vary in the ICU, making it essential to individualize comfort care with a patient-centered algorithm. Some patients who are conscious are able to report dyspnea, but others being withdrawn from the ventilator are critically ill, cognitively impaired, or unconscious and unable to self-report dyspnea. These patients may or may not be able to experience respiratory distress depending on the severity of unconsciousness.[2] The ability to experience unrelieved dyspnea continues until death. These patients near death are vulnerable to be under-recognized and under-treated for respiratory distress. Conversely, a patient runs the risk of being over-treated, which leads to oversedation and unintentional acceleration of death.[3] Unanticipated respiratory distress is a common complication of CE and one of the most challenging symptoms for health care providers to control for their patients. This can be an extremely stressful experience for patients, as well as their families and the health care team.

Without a standardized approach or guidelines, bedside nurses of a 24-bed medical intensive care unit (MICU) identified uncertainty about the best practice for CE. Team members struggled with how to implement evidence-based interventions while personalizing care for each patient's symptoms. Through an interdisciplinary unit leadership team vote, CE was chosen as a unit performance improvement project. The primary goal included improving the ventilator weaning process for patients and staff at EOL. Through an interdisciplinary team approach, an algorithm was established to implement the appropriate patient care before and during the terminal ventilator withdrawal, using the Respiratory Distress Observation Scale (RDOS) (**Fig. 1**). After unit-specific education on the correct use of RDOS in conjunction with the CE algorithm was completed, implementation of RDOS was started with EOL patients, along with collecting RDOS scores as a pilot study for 2 months. Comparison of N = 58 patients (26 patients pre-RDOS use and 32 patients using RDOS) took into consideration if there were any differences with the MICU population pre-RDOS implementation. Demographic data were similar between both groups, including comparable Apache IV scores, as well as time from extubation to death, and hospital length of stay. The results reflected the RDOS median score of 3.5 before extubation, RDOS median score of 2 at time of extubation, and RDOS median score of 2 after extubation with RDOS goal of less than 4. Preimplementation and postimplementation surveys also revealed evidence of decreased patient distress after CE and reduction of anxiety among staff during the process. Both survey results and RDOS data demonstrated the achievement of project goals. Implementation of pilot into practice was determined by interdisciplinary approval, and is system-wide today. This process has been shared locally, regionally, and nationally for others to implement; as it is important for all nurses caring for EOL, palliative patients to have the same resources to ensure quality of care and best outcomes for their patients and their families.

DISCUSSION

The RDOS is an objective assessment that guides the CE process. It is an objective tool used to assess the nonverbal, adult patient for the presence and intensity of

Respiratory Distress Observation Scale © (Margaret L. Campbell, PhD, RN 2/19/09)

Variable	0 points	1 point	2 points	Total
Heart rate per minute	<90 beats	90-109 beats	≥110 beats	
Respiratory rate per minute	≤18 breaths	19-30 breaths	>30 breaths	
Restlessness: non-purposeful movements	None	Occasional, slight movements	Frequent movements	
Paradoxical breathing pattern: abdomen moves in on inspiration	None		Present	
Accessory muscle use: rise in clavicle during inspiration	None	Slight rise	Pronounced rise	
Grunting at end-expiration: guttural sound	None		Present	
Nasal flaring: involuntary movement of nares	None		Present	
Look of fear	None		Eyes wide open, facial muscles tense, brow furrowed, mouth open, teeth together	
Total				

Instruction for use:
1. RDOS is not a substitute for patient self-report if able.
2. RDOS is an adult assessment tool.
3. RDOS cannot be used when the patient is paralyzed with a neuromuscular blocking agent.
4. RDOS is not valid in bulbar ALS or quadriplegia.
5. Count respiratory and heart rates for one-minute; auscultate if necessary.
6. Grunting may be audible with intubated patients on auscultation.
7. Fearful facial expressions:

Fig. 1. The Respiratory Distress Observation Scale (RDOS©) is an eight-item ordinal scale to measure the presence and intensity of respiratory distress in adults. It is intended for assessing the presence and intensity of respiratory distress when a patient is unable to report dyspnea. Each parameter is scored from 0 to 2 points and the points are summed. Scale scores range from 0 signifying no distress to 16 signifying the most severe distress. The scale was developed from a biobehavioral framework by Dr Margaret L. Campbell.[4,5] Psychometric testing for inter-rater and scale reliability as well as construct, convergent, and discriminant validity has been done. The internal consistency (α) across studies has ranged 0.64 to 0.86.[6] Inter-rater reliability was perfect between nurse data collectors (r = 1.0). Construct validity was established through correlation with hypoxemia, and use of oxygen.[6,7] Convergent validity was established through comparison with dyspnea self-report.[7] Discriminant validity was established with comparisons of RDOS from COPD patients with dyspnea to patients with acute pain and healthy volunteers.[7] Receiver Operating Curve analysis determined RDOS score 0 to 2 suggests no respiratory distress, score = 3 signifies mild, scores 4 to 6 signifies moderate, and ≥7 represents severe distress.[3,8] Similar psychometrics have been identified by other investigators.[9,10] RDOS is not valid with neonates, young children, patients with cervical spinal cord lesions producing quadriplegia nor with patients with bulbar amyotrophic lateral sclerosis. RDOS has clinical utility for assessing respiratory distress across settings of care including the ICU.[2] RDOS has research utility as a dependent measure in efficacy trials.[2,11] RDOS is in clinical use in more than 60 sites in the United States and in 11 countries. Translations have been done into French, Dutch, Chinese, Italian, Tamil, and Greek. For permission to use the RDOS, contact Dr Campbell at m.campbell@wayne.edu.

respiratory distress. There are 8 variables with numeric values, which are totaled together to obtain the RDOS score. Scale scores can vary from 0 indicating no distress to 16 indicating the most severe distress. The goal is a score less than 4. RDOS validates the need for comfort measures or medication to decrease respiratory distress, and/or pain. Dr Margaret Campbell, a nurse scientist at Wayne State University in Detroit, Michigan, developed the evidence-based tool. Summarization of the reliability and validity of the RDOS tool is under **Fig. 1.** Dr Campbell's clinical research and creation of this nurse-driven tool has allowed critical care teams to improve on the comfort of the dying patient. One of Campbell's studies was a 2-group observational design trialing a terminal ventilator withdrawal algorithm done in 2 MICUs. All control patients in one MICU underwent a one-step terminal extubation process under unstandardized care, whereas the nurses and respiratory therapists were educated on an algorithm that was used for an intervention group in another MICU.[2] The intervention group demonstrated no incidences of postextubation stridor, as well as reports of greater respiratory comfort.[2] Differences in medication use were noted with lorazepam being used more in the control group, whereas morphine use was recommended in the algorithm in the interventional group.[2] Using the RDOS in conjunction with guidelines and an algorithm can aid in the process of withdrawing life-sustaining measures in the clinical setting (**Figs. 2** and **3**).

The CE algorithm and the RDOS tool together allow nurses to follow clearly delineated chronologic steps for ease of use and efficiency. When further life-sustaining treatment is determined futile, and/or is no longer achieving the patient and family's goals of care, the family may choose to discontinue further treatment. Preparation

POPULATION: Comfort care and/or hospice patients only
PURPOSE: To standardize patient care at the end-of-life; to standardize the approach to compassionate extubation using Respiratory Distress Observation Scale (RDOS)

Provider Checklist
1. Comfort care power plan is for COMFORT CARE and/or HOSPICE patients ONLY.
2. Clarify and document goals of care, code status and end-of-life priorities.
3. Consider a consult to: social work for hospice referral, pastoral care for existential distress and/or palliative care for severe psychosocial distress or refractory symptoms.
4. Reconcile all active orders. Discontinue orders that are not comfort oriented (ie. labs, radiology studies, finger stick glucose checks, telemetry, monitors, BP cuffs, pulse oximetry, SCDs, invasive monitoring, etc).
5. Discontinue all medications that are not contributing to comfort (ie. statins, subcutaneous heparin, multivitamins).
6. Consider discontinuing artificial nutrition and intravenous hydration if consistent with goals of care.
7. Deactivate defibrillator and/or consider using magnet to disable defibrillator function (contact manufacturer or cardiology).
8. Think about strategy for treating symptoms during palliation using appropriate assessment scale (numeric rating system, etc) for patients who can self-report or RDOS scale for those who cannot self-report. (see interdisciplinary huddle)

Nursing Checklist
1. Assess patient comfort q 15-30 minutes initially for: pain, dyspnea, secretions, delirium/agitation, anxiety, nausea/vomiting, constipation and fever. Utilize appropriate assessment scales (numeric rating system, etc) to evaluate for presence of symptoms. In patients who cannot self-report, use RDOS scale.
2. Once comfort achieved assess above symptoms q1hr and PRN.
3. Check vital signs (BP, HR, RR, Temp) q 24hrs or q shift and PRN. Remove external monitoring devices not necessary for comfort (ie. BP cuff, SCDs, telemetry leads).
4. Silence any room (monitor, bed) alarms.
5. Oral care daily and PRN for comfort (ie. oral suction only for comfort). Turn and position PRN for comfort (ie. reposition patient's head to minimize noisy respirations)
6. Consider a fan for relief of dyspnea.
7. Try to get a private room. Identify room as comfort care.
8. Liberalize visitation and prepare the room for family/friends.
9. Assess family for bereavement needs and/or funeral arrangements, consider a consult to SW or Pastoral Care or discuss these needs with hospice (if hospice is involved in patient's care).
10. Offer bereavement cart

Interdisciplinary Huddle
1. Discuss anticipated severity of symptoms and strategy for symptom management using RDOS scale with a goal < 4
2. If present, review sequence of discontinuing life sustaining therapies (IABP, ECMO, pressors, AICD/pacer, mechanical ventilation).
3. Discuss likely disposition based on anticipated time to death (keep in ICU, transfer to hospice unit, floor bed, or home. * If patient intubated with plans to extubate and transfer to CCHS inpatient hospice unit (6D), may consider extubating after transfers to hospice unit)

Withdrawal of life support
1. Titrate medications to maintain RDOS < 4
2. Discontinue additional life sustaining interventions (pressors, IABP, ECMO, mechanical ventilation, HFNC/NIPPV etc.) in a stepwise manner as discussed in huddle
3. For removal of NIPPV/HFNC: if on high settings and/or FiO2 consider reducing settings in a stepwise manner and completely remove when patient appears comfortable and RDOS at goal
4. For removal of mechanical ventilation: reduce vent settings in a stepwise manner over a period of 15-30 minutes to PS 5, PEEP 0 and 21% FiO2. Extubate to room air when patient appears comfortable and RDOS at goal. *May consider extubation to NIPPV/O2 depending on expected outcomes and patient/family goals*
5. For discontinuation of IABP: place on 1:3, or stand-by depending on family request and leave in place until after patient expires.
6. For discontinuation of percutaneous ventricular assist devices: when patient comfortable and RDOS at goal, a left ventricular device should be turned off and pulled out of the ventricle and into the aorta. Right ventricular assist device should be turned off and moved out of the ventricle and into the IVC. Neither device (right or left) should be kept across a valve when the device is off. Leave cannula in place until after patient expires.
7. For discontinuation of ECMO: weaning varies depending of type of ECMO (VV, AV) support and is on case-by-case basis. Seek provider input and discuss plan in interdisciplinary huddle. Leave cannula in place until after patient expires.

Fig. 2. Comfort care at end-of-life for ICU inpatient care guideline.

ICU Symptom Management
Order medications using ICU Comfort Care power plan MD5595
For all medications, consider consultation with pharmacist for
assistance with dosing and calculations.

1. Pain/Dyspnea
❖ Consider most appropriate route of administration and need for
  bolus vs infusion based on anticipated severity of symptoms.
❖ If patient on current opioid therapy and is comfortable, continue
  current regimen and titrate as needed.
❖ If anxiety is contributing to respiratory distress, consider
  benzodiazepine (see anxiety).

SL opioids:
❖ **PRN dosing:**
  • Morphine Liquid Concentrate 20mg/ml (Roxanol) 5mg SL q1
    hr prn RDOS ≥ 4. If patient symptomatic after 2 doses, contact
    provider to increase PRN dose by 50% for mild-moderate
    symptoms and 100% for severe symptoms.
❖ **PRN dosing:**
  • OxyCODone 20mg/ml (OxyFast) Liquid Concentrate 5mg SL
    q 1hr prn RDOS ≥ 4 If patient symptomatic after 2 doses,
    contact provider to increase PRN dose by 50% for mild-
    moderate symptoms and 100% for severe symptoms.

IV Opioids/Benzodiazepine:
MORPHINE
❖ **PRN dosing:**
  • Initiate 2mg IV bolus every 10 minutes PRN for RDOS ≥ 4. If
    patient symptomatic after 2 doses, contact provider to increase
    PRN dose by 50% for mild-moderate symptoms and 100% for
    severe symptoms. *If 2 or more boluses are required per hour*
    for 2 consecutive hours, consider starting a continuous
    infusion.
  • Determine start rate by adding up the total boluses administered
    during the weaning process and divide by 2 to determine initial
    hourly dose and then refer to the titration chart for corresponding
    bolus and titration.
❖ **On regularly scheduled intermittent opioid therapy and**
  requires infusion:
  • Calculate the total daily dose used in the previous 24 hours
    (include both IV and PO equivalents), convert to IV equivalents
    and divide by 24 to determine initial hourly rate. Then refer to
    titration chart for corresponding bolus and titration.
❖ **On continuous opioid therapy:**
  • If RDOS <4, maintain IV infusion at current rate. If RDOS not at
    goal, bolus every 10 minutes PRN until comfortable and follow
    titration chart.
  • *If 2 or more boluses are required per hour, increase infusion*
    rate per titration chart. Do NOT increase infusion rate more
    frequently than every 1 hour.

Morphine Infusion and Bolus Titration Chart

Infusion Rate	PRN Bolus Dose
1mg/hr	2mg every 10 mins
2mg/hr	2mg every 10 mins
3mg/hr	2mg every 10 mins
5mg/hr	3mg every 10 mins
8mg/hr	4mg every 10 mins
12mg/hr	6mg every 10 mins
16mg/hr	8mg every 10 mins
20mg/hr	10mg every 10 mins
26mg/hr	15mg every 10 mins

Fig. 2. (continued)

for withdrawal of life-sustaining measures begins with communication between the
patient/family and the ICU team using a family/patient-centered care approach. Patients (when appropriate) and family members should be informed about the process,
the role of each team member, and what to expect during the dying process. Vital
signs, changes in appearance, signs of distress, and how the distress will be assessed
and treated using RDOS need to be explained. The family should be informed that the
time between CE and death is variable for each patient and can be difficult to predict
by the health care team. Hospital spiritual/pastoral care, or patient's own spiritual

FENTANYL

❖ **PRN dosing:**

- Initiate 25mcg IV bolus every 10 minutes PRN. If patient symptomatic after 2 doses, contact provider to increase PRN dose by 50% for mild-moderate symptoms and 100% for severe symptoms. *If 2 or more boluses are required per hour for 2 consecutive hours, consider starting a continuous infusion.*
- Determine start rate by adding up the total boluses administered during the weaning process and divide by 2 to determine initial hourly dose and then refer to the titration chart for corresponding bolus and titration.

❖ **On regularly scheduled intermittent opioid therapy and requires infusion:**

- Calculate the total daily dose used in the previous 24 hours (include both IV and PO equivalents), convert to IV equivalents and divide by 24 to determine initial hourly rate. Then refer to titration chart for corresponding bolus and titration.

❖ **On continuous opioid therapy :**

- If RDOS < 4, maintain IV infusion at current rate. If RDOS not at goal, bolus every 10 minutes PRN until comfortable and follow titration chart.
- *If 2 or more boluses are required per hour, increase infusion rate per titration chart. Do NOT increase infusion rate more frequently than every 1 hour.*

MIDAZOLAM

❖ **PRN dosing:**

- Initiate Midazolam 1mg IV bolus q 1 hr prn. If patient symptomatic after 2 doses, contact provider to increase PRN dose by 50% for mild-moderate symptoms and 100% for severe symptoms. *If boluses are not achieving patient comfort consider starting a midazolam infusion.*
- Begin infusion at 1mg/hr and titrate to RDOS < 4 using the titration chart.

❖ **On regularly scheduled intermittent benzodiazepine and requires infusion:**

- Calculate the total daily dose used in the previous 24 hours (include both PO and IV equivalents), convert to IV equivalents and divide by 24 to determine initial hourly rate. Then refer to titration chart for corresponding bolus and titration.

❖ **On continuous benzodiazepine therapy:**

- If RDOS < 4, maintain IV infusion at current rate. If RDOS not at goal, bolus every 10 minutes PRN until comfortable and follow titration chart.
- *If 2 or more boluses are required per hour, increase infusion rate per titration chart. Do NOT increase infusion rate more frequently than every 1 hour.*

Fentanyl Infusion and Bolus Titration Chart

Infusion Rate	PRN Bolus Dose
25mcg/hr	25mcg every 10 mins
50mcg/hr	25mcg every 10 mins
75mcg/hr	50mcg every 10 mins
100mcg/hr	50mcg every 10 mins
125mcg/hr	75mcg every 10 mins
150mcg/hr	75mcg every 10 mins
200mcg/hr	100mcg every 10 mins

Midazolam Titration Chart

Infusion Rate	PRN Bolus Dose
1mg/hr	1mg every 10 mins
2mg/hr	1mg every 10 mins
3mg/hr	1mg every 10 mins
4mg/hr	2mg every 10 mins
6mg/hr	2mg every 10 mins
8mg/hr	3mg every 10 mins
10mg/hr	3mg every 10 mins
12mg/hr	3mg every 10 mins

Fig. 2. (continued)

leader, and social work should be offered to be present during EOL discussions.[12] Identifying the patient/family goals and educating the patient/family are ongoing throughout the process and can be done by all members of the ICU team. Promoting a peaceful and calm environment is essential. Nurses can promote this by securing a private room, liberalizing visiting hours, dimming lights, and suspending alarms. An inconspicuous object can be placed on the door or curtain signaling to all unit staff that comfort care and CE are in progress to allow a quiet and respectful atmosphere.

An interdisciplinary huddle is essential to discuss and compose an individualized plan of care before CE for each patient. Orders for laboratories, tests, nonessential medications, invasive monitoring, sequential compression devices (SCDs), telemetry, monitors,

PROPOFOL

❖ **Should be reserved for severe myoclonus refractory to traditional treatment**

❖ Initiate as a continuous IV infusion at 5mcg/kg/minute IV and titrate every 5 mins as needed in increments of 5mcg/kg/min. Notify if dose exceeds 80mcg/kg/min. Titrate to RDOS <4.

❖ If patient is on propofol for general sedation and has no myoclonus transition to alternative agent for weaning.

Symptom Management – Continued from Page 1

2. Anxiety

❖ PRN dosing:

- Lorazepam 1mg PO/IV q 1 hr prn RDOS ≥ 4. If patient symptomatic after 2 doses, contact provider to increase PRN dose by 50% for mild-moderate symptoms and 100% for severe symptoms.
- Midazolam 1mg IV q 1 hr PRN RDOS ≥ 4. If patient symptomatic after 2 doses, contact provider to increase PRN dose by 50% for mild-moderate symptoms and 100% for severe symptoms.

3. Nausea and Vomiting

❖ Ondansetron disintegrating tablet 4mg PO q 6 hrs prn
❖ Ondansetron 4mg IV q 6 hrs prn
❖ Prochlorperazine 10mg IV q 6 hrs prn
❖ Prochlorperazine 10mg PO q 6 hrs prn

4. Secretions

❖ Glycopyrrolate 0.2mg IV q 2 hrs prn
❖ Hyoscyamine 0.125mg sublingual q 4 hrs prn (max daily dose 1.5mg)
❖ Atropine 1 drop (1% ophthalmic solution) sublingual q 2 hrs prn
❖ Scopolamine 1.5mg transdermal patch q 72 hrs

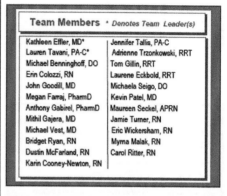

Equianalgesic Conversion of Opioids

Drug	SQ/IV Dose	Oral Dose
Morphine	10mg	30mg
Oxycodone	---	20mg
Hydromorphone	1.5mg	7.5mg
Fentanyl	100mcg (single dose)	---

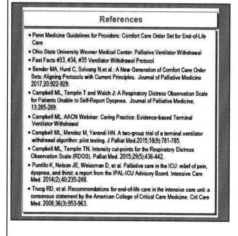

Team Members • *Denotes Team Leader(s)*

Kathleen Effler, MD*	Jennifer Tallis, PA-C
Lauren Tavani, PA-C*	Adrienne Trzonkowski, RRT
Michael Benninghoff, DO	Tom Gillin, RRT
Erin Colozzi, RN	Laurene Eckbold, RRT
John Goodill, MD	Michaela Seigo, DO
Megan Farraj, PharmD	Kevin Patel, MD
Anthony Gabirel, PharmD	Maureen Seckel, APRN
Mithil Gajera, MD	Jamie Turner, RN
Michael Vest, MD	Eric Wickersham, RN
Bridget Ryan, RN	Myrna Malak, RN
Dustin McFarland, RN	Carol Ritter, RN
Karin Cooney-Newton, RN	

References

- Penn Medicine Guidelines for Providers: Comfort Care Order Set for End-of-Life Care
- Ohio State University Wexner Medical Center: Palliative Ventilator Withdrawal
- Fast Facts #33, #34, #35 Ventilator Withdrawal Protocol
- Bender MA, Hurd C, Solvang N,et al.: A New Generation of Comfort Care Order Sets: Aligning Protocols with Current Principles. Journal of Palliative Medicine 2017;20:922-929.
- Campbell ML, Templin T and Walch J: A Respiratory Distress Observation Scale for Patients Unable to Self-Report Dyspnea. Journal of Palliative Medicine; 13:285-289.
- Campbell ML. AACN Webinar: Caring Practice: Evidence-based Terminal Ventilator Withdrawal
- Campbell ML, Mendez M, Yarandi HN. A two-group trial of a terminal ventilator withdrawal algorithm: pilot testing. J Palliat Med.2015;18(9):781-785.
- Campbell ML, Templin TN. Intensity cut-points for the Respiratory Distress Observation Scale (RDOS). Palliat Med. 2015;29(5):436-442.
- Puntillo K, Nelson JE, Weissman D, et al. Palliative care in the ICU: relief of pain, dyspnea, and thirst: a report from the IPAL-ICU Advisory Board. Intensive Care Med. 2014;2(2);40:235-248.
- Truog RD, et al. Recommendations for end-of-life care in the intensive care unit: a consensus statement by the American College of Critical Care Medicine. Crit Care Med. 2008;36(3):953-963.

Fig. 2. (continued)

and pulse oximetry are discontinued. Removal of naso-gastric tube/oral gastric tube (NGT/OGT), intravenous (IV) fluids, tube feeding, and foley catheter is done if interfering with the patient's comfort. In the huddle, a discussion of how much ventilator support the patient is currently receiving and if prior spontaneous breathing trial attempts took place should be reviewed. Other relative support needs to be evaluated too. Is the patient on any vasopressors and at what rate? This allows the team to anticipate possible distress and gives an idea of how imminent death will be after extubation.[13] Discussion of the patient's current medications occurs during the huddle with the recommendation

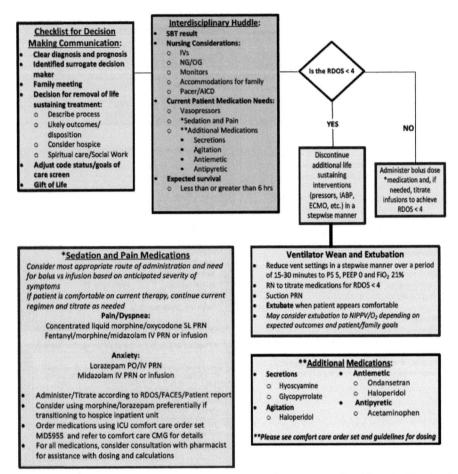

Checklist for Decision Making Communication:
- Clear diagnosis and prognosis
- Identified surrogate decision maker
- Family meeting
- Decision for removal of life sustaining treatment:
  ○ Describe process
  ○ Likely outcomes/disposition
  ○ Consider hospice
  ○ Spiritual care/Social Work
- Adjust code status/goals of care screen
- Gift of Life

Interdisciplinary Huddle:
- SBT result
- Nursing Considerations:
  ○ IVs
  ○ NG/OG
  ○ Monitors
  ○ Accommodations for family
  ○ Pacer/AICD
- Current Patient Medication Needs:
  ○ Vasopressors
  ○ *Sedation and Pain
  ○ **Additional Medications
    ▪ Secretions
    ▪ Agitation
    ▪ Antiemetic
    ▪ Antipyretic
- Expected survival
  ○ Less than or greater than 6 hrs

Is the RDOS < 4

YES   NO

Discontinue additional life sustaining interventions (pressors, IABP, ECMO, etc.) in a stepwise manner

Administer bolus dose *medication and, if needed, titrate infusions to achieve RDOS < 4

*Sedation and Pain Medications
Consider most appropriate route of administration and need for bolus vs infusion based on anticipated severity of symptoms
If patient is comfortable on current therapy, continue current regimen and titrate as needed
Pain/Dyspnea:
Concentrated liquid morphine/oxycodone SL PRN
Fentanyl/morphine/midazolam IV PRN or infusion

Anxiety:
Lorazepam PO/IV PRN
Midazolam IV PRN or infusion

- Administer/Titrate according to RDOS/FACES/Patient report
- Consider using morphine/lorazepam preferentially if transitioning to hospice inpatient unit
- Order medications using ICU comfort care order set MD5955 and refer to comfort care CMG for details
- For all medications, consider consultation with pharmacist for assistance with dosing and calculations

Ventilator Wean and Extubation
- Reduce vent settings in a stepwise manner over a period of 15-30 minutes to PS 5, PEEP 0 and FiO$_2$ 21%
- RN to titrate medications for RDOS < 4
- Suction PRN
- Extubate when patient appears comfortable
- *May consider extubation to NIPPV/O$_2$ depending on expected outcomes and patient/family goals*

**Additional Medications:
- Secretions
  ○ Hyoscyamine
  ○ Glycopyrrolate
- Agitation
  ○ Haloperidol
- Antiemetic
  ○ Ondansetran
  ○ Haloperidol
- Antipyretic
  ○ Acetaminophen

**Please see comfort care order set and guidelines for dosing

Fig. 3. Comfort care ICU inpatient—flow diagram for CE care algorithm (quick visual resource).

that if the patient is already comfortable on an opioid and/or sedative, these medications should be continued at those doses during CE.[12] If the patient is on propofol for general sedation and has no myoclonus, transitioning to an alternative agent before CE should be completed.[14] Propofol should be reserved for severe myoclonus refractory to traditional treatment. For opioid-naïve patients, morphine is the initial opioid of choice for pain and/or dyspnea.[12,15] Morphine is the evidence-based choice for dyspnea relief.[15] According to Campbell, if morphine is effective alone, as it is with many patients, then sedation is not necessary. She suggests using lorazepam in addition if there is a need to frequently bolus with morphine.[15] Downar and colleagues recommend that sedation should only be used once pain and dyspnea are effectively treated with opioids (2016).[12] Additional medications are ordered in anticipation of agitation, secretions, and antiemetic, and antipyretic needs.

It is important to note the guidelines and algorithms as support during the process of CE. Each event must be individualized to each patient, noting his or her specific needs and prioritizing comfort at all times. The use of the RDOS will validate the need for the patient to receive medication for comfort before moving on to the next step. If the

RDOS is not less than 4, premedicate with a bolus of morphine via IV push or continuous infusion. RDOS will be reassessed every 10 minutes, rebolusing, if necessary, until RDOS less than 4.[14] If the patient is not on a morphine infusion and 2 or more boluses are required per hour for 2 consecutive hours, starting a continuous infusion is warranted. Determine the starting infusion rate of the morphine drip by adding the total boluses administered during the weaning process and dividing by 2 to determine the initial hourly dose and then refer to the titration chart in **Fig. 2**.[14,15] When the RDOS score is less than 4, the patient is ready for the next step.

CE steps:

- If planning allows 24-hour advance notice:
  - Diurese if the patient is fluid overloaded and has the presence of wet lung sounds to reduce the volume of postextubation secretions
  - Restrict fluid intake
  - Check for cuff leak and if no cuff leak, reduce the risk for postextubation stridor-begin
    Dexamethasone 4 mg IV q 6- reduces the risk of postextubation stridor[15]
- Determine the need for premedication using RDOS to validate. RDOS less than 4 is GOAL
- If RDOS is not less than 4, administer a bolus dose of morphine and, if needed, titrate infusion to achieve RDOS less than 4 following guideline in **Fig. 2**
- If RDOS is less than 4, discontinue IV fluids and vasopressors to:
  - allow hypotension to occur naturally
  - reduce patient's consciousness and the ability to experience respiratory distress
  - allow for death before extubation
- Address patient/family goals and educate before discontinuation of vasopressors
- Discontinuation of vasopressors, Intra-aortic balloon pump (IABP), Extra-Corporeal Membrane Oxygenation (ECMO) should be in a stepwise manner
- Ventilator wean and extubation*
  - Reduce vent settings in a stepwise manner over a period of 15 to 30 minutes to Pressure support 5, positive end-expiratory pressure (PEEP) 0, and Fio_2 21% (this will be individualized)[14,15]
    1. Turn off PEEP[15]
    2. Wean Fio_2
    3. synchronized intermittent mandatory ventilation (SIMV)/pressure support ventilation (PSV)
    4. Wean PSV
    5. continuous positive airway pressure (CPAP) 0/PSV 5
    6. Determine need for postwithdrawal oxygen for comfort
       - SpO_2 less than 85% + RDOS greater than 4 – consider low flow O_2 via N/C[15]
       - O_2 is part of the family's discussed goals/request
       - Goal should be to extubate to room air[12]
    7. Extubate and turn off ventilator
       - Consider just turning off the ventilator and keeping the patient intubated if the patient did not pass the cuff-leak test to prevent postextubation stridor[15]
       - In a patient with COVID-19, the patient should remain intubated with a viral filter in place[16]

*Evaluate RDOS with every ventilator change: bolus with morphine if RDOS is not less than 4. The respiratory therapist and RN work together, in a stepwise manner to maintain a goal of RDOS less than 4. If further medication is not required, weaning steps can be done every 2 minutes[15]

- Emotional support and comfort for the family
  - Use of a bereavement cart, "comfort cart"—comfort care for family members providing beverages and snacks, which allows the family to stay in a room with the patient
  - Spiritual care/chaplain or priest
  - Education and review of any questions
  - Fingerprinting or printing of heart rhythm strip to save for memorabilia before CE
  - Use of a comfort blanket made by a volunteer
- Stridor occurs most often in the first hour after extubation
  - Risk factors
    - Traumatic intubation
    - History of self-extubation
    - Prolonged intubation
    - Elevated SAPS II (Simplified Acute Physiology Score)
  - Treatment
    - Racemic epinephrine aerosol, 2.5 mg in 3 cc normal saline
    - May need to repeat x1

SUMMARY

Using a standardized approach to CE and EOL care helps decrease stress for the patient, family, and the critical care team. An objective tool, such as the RDOS, guides the assessment, decision-making process, and appropriate medication administration to optimize patient comfort at EOL. The CE algorithm assists in selecting interventions to provide compassionate care for patients during the ventilator withdrawal period. Education of staff on the correct use of these tools, as well as clear communication and education with families on CE at EOL, is essential.

The CE guidelines and RDOS became especially valuable with the onset of the COVID-19 pandemic. This novel medical crisis has presented many challenges, weighing heavily on health care providers. One of the biggest challenges was the exclusion of family presence during hospitalization, especially for terminally ill patients. This unfathomable concept prompted nurses to be even more present for the EOL patient. Nurses became very creative using their personal cell phones and hospital-provided electronic devices to include family members virtually. The guideline, algorithm, and RDOS proved to be essential to ensure comfort and minimize anxiety and distress for the patients, families, and health care team.

Although EOL care is challenging and emotionally exhausting for all those involved, helping patients die peacefully can be as rewarding as saving a life. Thom Dick summarizes it best: "You're going to be there when a lot of people are born, and when a lot of people die. In most every culture, such moments are regarded sacred and private, made special by a divine presence. No one on Earth would be welcomed, but you're personally invited. What an honor that is."[17]

CLINICS CARE POINTS

- The ability to experience unrelieved dyspnea continues until death

- Patients near death are apt to be under-recognized and under-treated for respiratory distress
- Patients also run the risk of being over treated, which may lead to oversedation and unintentional acceleration of death
- EOL can be a stressful experience for patients, families, and the health care team
- Education and communication with the family help to identify the patient/family goals at EOL
- An interdisciplinary huddle is essential to compose an individualized plan of care before CE for each patient
- Goal score for RDOS is less than 4
- RDOS validates the need for comfort measures or medication to decrease respiratory distress while avoiding under-medicating or over-medicating patients
- RDOS is not valid with neonates, young children, patients with cervical spinal cord lesions producing quadriplegia nor with patients with bulbar amyotrophic lateral sclerosis
- Using RDOS, along with an algorithm optimizes comfort for the dying, adult, nonverbal patient
- Morphine is the evidence-based, recommended medication for the relief of dyspnea
- During CE, evaluation of RDOS is done with every ventilator change with RT and RN working together in a stepwise manner to maintain a goal of RDOS less than 4
- Consider turning off the ventilator and keeping the patient intubated if the patient did not pass the cuff-leak test to prevent postextubation stridor
- Stridor occurs most often in the first hour after extubation and is treated with racemic epinephrine
- Follow institutional guidelines to maintain safety for patients with COVID-19 at EOL; ex. COVID-19 patient remains intubated with viral filter in place

DISCLOSURE

The authors have nothing to disclose.

REFERENCES

1. Truog RD, Campbell ML, Curtis JR, et al. Recommendations for end-of-life in the intensive care unit: a consensus statement by the American College of Critical Care Medicine. Crit Care Med 2008;36:953–63.
2. Campbell ML, Yarandi HD, Mendez M. A two-group trial of a terminal ventilator withdrawal algorithm: pilot testing. J Palliat Med 2015;18(9):781–5.
3. Campbell ML, Templin TN. Intensity cut-points for the respiratory distress observation scale. Palliat Med 2015;29(5):436–42.
4. Campbell MK. Fear and pulmonary stress behaviors to an asphyxia threat across cognitive states. Res Nurs Health 2007;30(6):572–83.
5. Campbell ML. Respiratory distress: a model of responses and behaviors to an asphyxial threat for patients who are unable to self-report. Heart Lung 2008; 37(1):54–60.
6. Campbell ML, Templin T, Walch J. A respiratory distress observation scale for patients unable to self-report dyspnea. J Palliat Med 2010;13(3):285–90.
7. Campbell ML. Psychometric testing of a respiratory distress observation scale. J Palliat Med 2008;11(1):44–50.

8. Campbell ML, Kero KK, Templin TN. Mild, moderate, and severe intensity cut-points for the respiratory distress observation scale. Heart Lung 2017; 46(1):14–7.
9. Chan YH, Wu HS, Yen CC, et al. Psychometric evaluation of the Chinese respiratory distress observation scale on critically ill patients with Cardiopulmonary Diseases. J Nurs Res 2018;26(5):340–7.
10. Zhuang Q, Yang GM, Neo SH, et al. Validity, reliability and diagnostic accuracy of the respiratory distress observation scale for assessment of dyspnea in adult palliative care patients. J Pain Symptom Manage 2018;57(2):304–10.
11. Campbell ML, Yarandi H, Dove-Medows E. Oxygen is nonbeneficial for most patients who are near death. J Pain Symptom Manage 2013;45(3):517–23.
12. Downar J, Delaney JW, Hawryluck L, et al. Guidelines for the withdrawal of life-sustaining measures. Intensive Care Med 2016;42:1003–17.
13. Long AC, Muni S, Treece PD, et al. Time to death after terminal withdrawal of mechanical ventilation: specific respiratory and physiologic parameters may inform physician predictions. J Palliat Med 2015;18(12):1040–7.
14. Effler, et al. Christiana care management, comfort care at end-of-life for ICU inpatient care guideline. 2020.
15. Campbell ML. American Association of Critical- Care Nurses (AACN) Webinar: caring practice: evidence-based terminal ventilator withdrawal. 2016.
16. Dick T. People Care Perspectives & Practices for Professional Caregivers. 3rd Edition. HMP Publishing; 2019.
17. Top 15 quotes about Nursing that will empower you. In: Nursing file. 2015. Available at: http://nursinglife,com. Accessed July 30, 2021.

Serious Illness Discussion in Palliative Care—A Case Study Approach in an African American Patient with Cancer

Deborah Russell, MSN, FNP-BC, APRN-NP, ACHPN[a,*],
Jo Clarke, DNP, ANP-BC, NP-C, ACNP-BC, APRN-CNP, AOCNP[b],
Lynne Brophy, MSN, PMGT-BC, APRN-CNS, AOCN[c],
Michele L. Weber, DNP, RN, APRN-CNS, APRN-NP, CCRN, CCNS, OCN, AOCNS[d]

KEYWORDS

- People of color - African Americans - Serious illness conversations
- Advanced care planning - End of life - Documentation - Goal concordant care
- Advanced cancer patients

KEY POINTS

- Serious illness conversation should start when a serious illness is diagnosed, not near the time of death. Documentation using the Advance Care Planning format should occur during the illness trajectory and updated at each encounter.
- Nurses are an invaluable resource in gathering cultural and spiritual beliefs during these conversations, especially with the African American population.
- Serious illness conversations should be documented using a template across the illness trajectory in a way that can be easily identified by colleagues working in all health care settings (ICU, clinic, etc)

INTRODUCTION

Advancements in cancer care extend life but have created a difficult juncture between medical futility and quality of life.[1] Early discussions of patient wishes may inform

[a] Department of Palliative Medicine, Arthur G. James Hospital and Richard J. Solove Research Institute, The Ohio State University Wexner Medical Center, 1581 Dodd Drive, 5th Floor McCampbell Hall, Columbus, OH 43210 USA; [b] Department of Internal Medicine, Division of Medical Oncology, Arthur G. James Hospital and Richard J. Solove Research Institute, The Ohio State University Wexner Medical Center, 460 West 10th Avenue, Columbus, OH 43210, USA; [c] The Ohio State University Cancer Comprehensive Center and Richard J. Solove Research Institute, The Ohio State University, Stefanie Spielman Comprehensive Breast Center, Administration – Room 2040, 1145, Olentangy River Road, Columbus, OH 43212, USA; [d] Arthur G. James Hospital and Richard J. Solove Research Institute, The Ohio State University Wexner Medical Center, 460 West 10th Avenue, Columbus, OH 43210, USA
* Corresponding author.
E-mail address: Deborah.russell@osumc.edu

Crit Care Nurs Clin N Am 34 (2022) 79–90
https://doi.org/10.1016/j.cnc.2021.11.006
0899-5885/22/© 2021 Elsevier Inc. All rights reserved.
ccnursing.theclinics.com

treatment decisions and, in some cases, prevent futile care. Knowing when to begin these discussions can be difficult. Estimation of prognosis has improved because of qualitative and quantitative methods used in the cancer population. One tool that can be used is the Palliative Performance Scale (PPS). This scale has shown potential for prognosticating survival.[2] This scale has 5 domains: ambulation, activity, evidence of disease, self-care, and level of consciousness. Despite this increased insight, initial serious illness conversations (SICs) commonly occur when a patient is in a crisis or requires intensive care unit (ICU) admission. Prioritizing earlier SICs that include the patient's preferred decision makers can promote the provision of goal concordant care that aligns with the patient and family's values and cultural beliefs as well as the avoidance of unnecessary overtreatment or undertreatment. African American culture and beliefs present unique considerations in conducting SICs. Ideally, SICs should begin when or shortly after the diagnosis of serious illness with a poor prognosis. The conversation can continue at future inpatient and outpatient encounters. These ongoing conversations require accessible and easily retrievable documentation by all health care team members. This article will address how a nurse might facilitate and participate in these conversations using a case study to illustrate this process.

BACKGROUND AND SIGNIFICANCE

Hospitalized patients with advanced cancer and their families are frequently inadequately informed or educated about their cancer diagnosis, prognosis, and care options unless a crisis occurs. This limits them from making educated reasonable decisions concerning their end of life, including the decision to pursue palliative care.[3,4] Many patients die without the benefit of aligning their end-of-life preferences with the plan of care or after having the discussions too late to realize any benefit.[5] Family members play an integral role in end-of-life decision-making, especially among African American patients.[6] However, many patients and family members experience poor communication with the health care team regarding end-of-life care.[6]

Unfortunately, the evidence reveals frequently, these discussions occur when there is little opportunity to pursue a reasonable and preferred end of life consistent with the patient's wishes because death is imminent.[7,8] Patients and their families are too often unaware of realistic options, or unprepared to adjust to predictable outcomes, or uninformed about helpful palliative interventions. Many are simply unprepared to die.[9,10] Candid, honest discussions can reduce symptom intensity, readmission rates, anxiety, length of stay, critical care intervention, decrease health care utilization at end of life, and increase hospice referrals.[3,11–15]

When cancer is diagnosed, there is an opportunity for the provider to explain current available therapies, rates of success, and plans if this therapy is not successful. This discussion should include the patient and his/her decision makers, usually a spouse or family member. By indicating palliative care will be a part of cancer treatment early in the illness trajectory after diagnosis, the provider can educate the patient and family that palliative care is critical to symptom management and not just reserved for consultation during the end of life. The provider may also introduce hospice as the preferred provider during the last 6 months of life. Introducing hospice as a usual form of care in the same manner as home care early in the disease process normalizes the transition to hospice if necessary. The documentation of this discussion is critical. The provider can end this discussion or care conference with a realistic summary of the goal of the patient's chosen cancer treatment, which may be cure, control of the cancer, or palliation. Initially, the patient and family may hope for the cancer to respond to conventional treatment.

Subsequent conversations between the provider, patient, and preferred decision-makers can occur at the patient's request or when cancer therapy is no longer achieving the initial goal of therapy. If palliative care providers have not been added to the treatment team previously, they can be consulted when disease control is no longer possible. The palliative care team can work with the patient and family to set goals, which often shifts to easing symptoms, addressing personal issues, or identifying where the patient wishes to die.[11,16] As cancer progresses, communication between the patient and the health care team offers an opportunity to prevent unwanted overtreatment or undertreatment and optimize concordance of care with the patient's wishes.[17,18] The critical care registered nurse (RN) is in the unique position to provide insight to other members of the health care team as decisions regarding health care interventions are being discussed. The Society of Critical Care Medicine ABCDEF Bundle[19] has as one of its pillars a focus on communication with the patient's family. The letter, "F" in the Bundle, focuses on family engagement and empowerment.[19] In critical care units that have completely implemented the ABCDEF Bundle, there was an association with a lower likelihood of 7 outcomes: hospital death within 7 days, next-day mechanical ventilation, coma, deliruim, physical restraint use, ICU readmission, and discharge to a facility other than home.[19] When operationalizing the ABCDEF Bundle in a medical intensive care setting, Weber and colleagues[20] encouraged the bedside critical care nurse to invite family members into daily multidisciplinary rounds. These bedside nurses also encourage family members to ask questions and provide information during rounds. The bedside nurses created an environment in daily multidisciplinary rounds when all members of the health care team were quiet and allowed family members to speak. Creating this quiet time allowed family members to inquire about the proposed plan of care for their family member.[20]The bedside nurses, also arranged daily telefamily calls to update family members who were not able to be present in-person at multidisciplinary rounds.[20] This focus on the family as part of the team may inform the health care team of the patient wishes regarding wanted or unwanted interventions. Ideally their health care can be adapted to the patient wishes and current circumstances to achieve desired and realistic care.[10]

SIC is the current term used to describe these conversations. SIC is an ongoing conversation starting early in the diagnosis of metastatic disease to educate, enlighten both the patient and provider, and offer the patient guidance, services, and resources.[4,18,21] A component of SIC is advanced care planning (ACP) that includes the discussion of designating a Health Care Power of Attorney (HCPOA) or writing a Living Will. ACP is a process through which decisions regarding future medical care are considered and communicated to medical providers to guide care of serious illness and capacity for decision making.[22] Each member of the health care team can contribute to this ongoing conversation. For example, the patient's nurse may have an informal discussion regarding the meaning of the word metastatic, side effects of treatments chosen, symptom management options, or what the patient fears. The nurse may discover the patient is resistant to pursuing palliative care or beginning hospice care because of the mistaken belief that it will cause an expedited death or result in withdrawal of symptom management measures. The findings of these conversations can make future conversations by any health care team member more efficient and productive for the patient and the entire health care team. The nurse is often the requestor of a case conference to discuss end-of-life wishes and is a key attendee of these meetings with the provider, patient, and decision-makers or family. The nurse is a key part of SIC. SIC is not a euphemism for absolute pursuit of hospice, or a "threatment" of impending death, but an open forum to clarify any patient, family, or provider misunderstandings and an opportunity to work toward desired and practical outcomes.

BARRIERS TO SICs

One predominant barrier to SIC is health care worker reluctance, inexperience, or lack of education in conducting SIC.[3,23,24] Hesitation to initiate a SIC is often based on discomfort with the topic, precise prognosis uncertainty, the perception that a less aggressive option is a failure, confusion over who should have the conversation, and fear of relinquishing patient hope.[3,23,25] The evidence discounts many of these assumptions, including the fear of diminishing patient hope or increasing patient distress.[4,14]

Though an exact prognosis may not be possible, as cancer progresses and functional status declines, the possibility of any improvement in quality of life with further treatment is remote. Previous studies have examined multiple methods of predicting prognosis with varying results. In one study, 343 experienced physicians were asked to give survival estimates for 468 terminally ill patients at the time of hospice referral. Although 20% gave accurate estimates for survival patients at the time of hospice referral, the majority of clinicians over estimated prognosis by a factor of 5.3.[26] Cancer survival can be considered by using 2 major categories: performance (functional) status, and signs and symptoms. One scale, the PPS offers a reliable and sensitive method of predicting life expectancy, which can be used by nurses to determine the urgency of SIC.[27] The PPS evaluates 5 domains: ambulation, activity, evidence of disease, self-care, and level of consciousness. The scores range in 10% increments from 10% to 100%. For example, a score of 0% indicates death, 10% indicates a bed-bound patient who is unable to do any activity and needs total assistance, and 100% indicates the patient can carry on normal activity and work.

Most patients and families are not familiar with medical terminology, and this may serve as a barrier to successful SICs. Owing to personal discomfort, trepidation, or misguided perceptions, the health care team may try to buffer the impact of unpleasant news by using medical terminology such as "progressing" or "palliative" that may confuse patients. These positive-sounding words may be misinterpreted as promising or reassuring for cure.[16] Lack of health literacy contributes to this misunderstanding.[1] Nurses can help to overcome these barriers by attending SICs whenever possible and after the conversation, providing clarification to the patient and participants. Educational programs such as Vital Talk (VT) seek to teach all members of the health care team how to phrase and conduct SICs.[28]

The case study presented in **Box 1** illustrates how culture is a crucial facet to consider when thinking about SIC serious illness discussion. In our case study, the patient is African American. People of color who have cancer are more likely to present at advanced stages of disease, are less likely to receive effective treatment including symptom control such as pain management, and are enrolled in hospice care at a lower rate.[29] Clinicians hypothesize that the reasons for these disparities may be multifactorial including patient-level or family-level, provider-level, and system-level factors.[29] An understanding of these factors may assist the clinician in offering more effective communication with people of color during SICs.

Patients and families of color may have beliefs that influence decision-making about medical care such as fatalistic thinking that terrible things are meant to happen, should be accepted, and are part of God's plan.[29] African Americans were more likely than other ethnic groups to view life support as absolutely required because of the belief that "only God should decide when it is time for death" and miracles are possible.[29] All patients may have preferences about who should help make decisions about care. In one study, most patients, irrespective of ethnicity, wished for bad news to be shared concurrently with themselves and their family members, rather than

Box 1
Case study

Introduction to the case study

Mrs X was a 54-year-old African American female Y.M. with a newly diagnosed squamous cell carcinoma (SCC) of the tongue. She had 2 adult children, a daughter and a son with autism who was not able to care for himself independently. She had a history of chronic pancreatitis secondary to alcohol use disorder and related chronic abdominal pain and a history of substance use disorder. When initially seen by Palliative Medicine, she was treatment naïve, actively using substances and due to start radiation later in the month. She was malnourished. A small-bore feeding tube was placed before radiation for enteral nutrition. She was not able to complete radiation because of transportation and multiple social issues. She relied on transportation provided through insurance for medical appointments and found it difficult to navigate this system. Mrs X was the primary caregiver for her daughter. Mrs X and her daughter lived with various relatives during the course of her illness. The patient was encouraged to make end-of-life plans during initial meetings with palliative care but did not wish to do so.

She was admitted to the hospital 4 times from the time of her cancer diagnosis to death for infection, pain, and failure to thrive. Each hospital stay was at least 2 to 3 weeks in duration. Hospital stays were complicated by pain control and malnutrition. Six months after initial diagnosis, she was found to have new lung metastasis due to SCC of the tongue. She underwent palliative radiation therapy of her tongue and struggled with pain control. Palliative care managed her pain. She formally designated her daughter as Healthcare Power of Attorney after several admissions. During her final hospitalization, 1 month after she was diagnosed with metastatic disease, she was admitted to the intensive care unit with a stroke, residual dysarthria, and sepsis. She was also found to have evidence of multiple previous embolic strokes. Unfortunately, Mrs X was unable to provide information about her care wishes to the critical care team during her ICU admission. As this was her first ICU admission, the critical care team relied on information from the medical record to guide them about her goals for her care.

Throughout all of her hospitalizations, there was no documentation of advance care planning or serious illness conversation until just before her death 9 months after diagnosis. By then, discussing her serious illness was limited to the very end-of-life care, and too late for her to choose how she wished to spend her final weeks of months because of her inability to communicate. The critical care team provided the standard of ICU care for Mrs X. Many of the interventions may have been uncomfortable and more invasive than Mrs X would have wanted. The ICU nurses provided ongoing support and encouragement to Mrs X and her family. They updated her family on the ICU interventions and plan of care for Mrs X. They sat with Mrs X's family in support and conversation to discover more about Mrs X as a person and mother. The ICU nurses guided these conversations to provide additional information to Mrs X's family and answered their questions. The ICU nurses provided 24-hour access to Mrs X per the unit's open visitation policy. This allowed Mrs X's family to visit as their schedules allowed. The ICU nurses facilitated the presence of Mrs X's family in daily multidisciplinary rounds. In this way, Mrs X's family was part of the health care team, part of decision-making, and part of the discussion when complex therapies and treatments were discussed. Based on Mrs X's condition, there came a time when the ICU nurses accompanied Mrs X's family members to formal goals of care meeting. A formal goals of care conversation was held between the ICU intensivist, the palliative care nurse practitioner, the ICU primary nurse, the patient, and the patient's adult daughter in the ICU, and the goals of care were changed to comfort care. Her daughter was her surrogate decision maker as Health Care Power of Attorney (HCPOA). Mrs X lacked medical capacity for decision making at this time. The presence of the ICU nurse at this goals of care meeting allowed the ICU nurses to be fully informed of the plan of care for Mrs X. It allowed the ICU nurses to support Mrs X's family as the focus of Mrs X's ICU care changed from aggressive interventions to comfort and support. The ICU nurses provided information to the health care team on which comfort measures had been effective to relieve Mrs X's symptoms during her current ICU stay. The ICU nurses advocated for the continuation of these interventions during the next phase of Mrs X's care. Mrs X died in the ICU with her family at the bedside a few days after the goals of care were changed.

individually.[29] Health literacy may affect decision-making. The findings from this study also revealed that African Americans were more likely than other ethnic and racial groups to believe that a living will precludes the patient from receiving cancer treatment. Subjects also believed that cardiopulmonary resuscitation (CPR) had a greater than 50% chance of being successful.[29] Minority groups are more likely to believe that hospice is an option only for patients who are going to die within a few days.[29] Jannalagadda's (2012) findings illustrate the need for assessment of patient and family wishes throughout the cancer trajectory.[29]

Cultural beliefs and other factors may influence ACP. ACP is substantially lower among African Americans than among Whites.[30] One study evaluated ACP interventions among older African Americans through improved focus on ACP. Engaging in ACP with this population is influenced by historical, personal, interpersonal, and system factors, mistrust in many factors including the health care system, access to care, religion and spirituality, family, community, and clinician interactions.[30] This large multisite study identified opportunities to improve ACP for African Americans, including a greater emphasis on the importance of these conversations with surrogates with or without legal documents, with providers, and flexibility in approaches to ACP based on individual preferences and increased education for facilitators of these discussions.

Clearly, lack of knowledge may drive decision-making. Kemp (2005) and Trip Reimer (1984) have suggested that the benefit of a full assessment of the patient's cultural beliefs before SIC or other nursing care takes place.[31,32] Kemp (2005) reminds the clinician, applying culture-specific knowledge to guide conversation, before assessing the individual and family results in stereotyping which is counterproductive.[31] Individuals and families make choices about their cultural practices. Tripp Reimer and others (1984) offer a simple set of questions that the nurse can ask to learn the patient and family's cultural beliefs before providing care or SIC.[32] These questions are summarized in **Box 2**. Our case study illustrates the importance of continued discussions through the cancer trajectory. Previous discussions can inform clinicians later in the illness trajectory or another setting (inpatient vs outpatient) who are planning SICs to continue ACP. Documentation of ACP and SICs is helpful to communicate what has been discussed to the entire medical team.

COMMUNICATION AND DOCUMENTATION

In addition to the need for improved communication between the health care team and the patient, there is also a need for improved communication between team members.[33,34] Health care teams value standardized workflows and SIC documentation.[33] Electronic medical record templates or "smart phrases" offer a format for consistent and easily retrievable SIC documentation.[34] These can be used to monitor quality, billing, and the occurrences of SIC. However, the primary advantage is improved clear communication between all health care team members.

Displays an example of a SIC template. The highlighted areas identify a list of choices the team member can simply click. This serves as a map to guide discussion and an efficient method to document **Box 3**.

There is little evidence of SIC education in initial or subsequent nurse education.[35] VT and The Serious Illness Conversation Program (SICP) (https://www.ariadnelabs.org/areas-of-work/serious-illness-care/) are 2 programs that have shown considerable success preparing productive SICs by health care team members.[28,36,37] Both programs incorporate role-play with simulated patients for real-time feedback, coaching, and strategies. These interactive training programs provide guidance and tools to

---

Box 2
Cultural assessment—a phased approach

First Phase—preliminary assessment

General physical and psychosocial assessment

Collection of cultural information: ethnicity, religion, patterns of health care, and general decision making; language, style of nonverbal and verbal communication, etiquette needs determined by culture such as touch, personal space, desired gender of caregivers, dietary needs, and so forth.

Sample questions:
- Would you describe yourself as a religious person and if so, what religion do you practice or believe in? What religious beliefs should I know about that might change your care?
- What do you think caused this to happen?
- Do you have an explanation for why it started when it did?
- What does this sickness do to you; how does it work?
- How severe do you feel this sickness is? Will it have a long or short duration?
- What kind of treatment do you think you should receive at this point?
- What are the most important results you hope to receive from this treatment?
- What problems has this sickness caused you or your family?
- What do you fear about this sickness?

Second phase—focused assessment to plan interventions and referrals

Is this condition good or bad?
- What have you been doing to treat this condition in the past and in the present?
- What do you plan to do in the future?
- How should a person who has this condition/problem act?
- How should one who has this condition be treated by family members?
- How do you spend your days at home and how do you wish to spend them?
- How has this illness affected your ability to do what you want each day?

Data from 32. Tripp-Reimer T, Brink PJ, Saunders JM. Cultural assessment: Content and process. Nursing Outlook, 1984;32:78-82; and 31. Kemp C. Culture issues in palliative care. Seminars in Oncology Nursing. 2005; 21(1):44-52. https://doi.org/10.1053/j.soncn.2004.10.0007

---

empower clinicians to communicate empathetically and effectively with patients and families about serious illnesses. One of the most challenging aspects of SIC is getting started.[28] VT and the SICP offer tools or guides for discussion with examples or recommendations of how to approach sensitive topics.[34] For example, the mnemonic "REMAP" stands for *R*eframe, *E*xpect emotion, *M*ap out the future, *A*lign with values, and *P*lan treatments (**Box 4**). This guides the team member to address patient values and offers structure to both SIC training and its actual implementation with patients and families.[28]

Conversation in the ICU can present a difficult challenge. If there have not been ongoing SICs with the patient and family, whether due to the unexpected patient decline, or simply failure to initiate, the conversation can be overwhelming. Without the preparation of previous SICs in preparation for the anticipated outcome of advanced cancer, the patient and family may be surprised to discover the seriousness of the condition, and possible imminent death. There is a growing position of avoidance of ICU admission for terminal cancer patients. The Centers for Medicare and Medicaid Services nationally monitors ICU admissions within 30 days of death, chemotherapy within 14 days of death, and admission to the hospital within 3 days of death (https//www.cms.gov). In the future, there may be reimbursement consequences for interventions deemed futile by payers. Critical care nurses recognize that there may be multiple reasons for an ICU admission for a patient with advanced

---

Box 3
Components of serious illness discussion documentation using a smart phrase

The patient and/or surrogate wishes to discuss their serious illness today.
  Advanced care provider (ACP) discussion
    I discussed with patient name and/or surrogate: ____insert name and relationship of
    surrogate___ their specific wishes for care in the event that they become seriously ill/
    worsens clinically. The patient and/or surrogate have an adequate understanding of the
    patient's current health status and the risk of serious illness or catastrophic event that
    could require life support. The patient holds cultural beliefs which will influence care
    decisions and are: _____.
  Is there concern regarding the patient's cognitive function or decision-making capacity?
    YES/NO:
    Will this clinician be surprised if this patient will be alive in 6 months? Yes/no
  Participants: participant choices
  Cancer type: list of types
  Intent of cancer treatment: curative, control vs palliative
  Long-term prognosis based on current health status: time choices or unknown
  Was this discussed with patient/surrogate?: yes/no
  Patient's understanding of prognosis: good/fare/poor/n/a
  General values/wishes if health worsens: list of commonly wished for situations, for example,
  be at home, be physically comfortable, and so forth.
  Serious Illness Conversation (SIC) Summary
    In the event of a serious and/or critical illness, the patient expresses the following
    preferences for care *based on their values.*
  Surrogate Decision-Maker(s): (NOTE: A surrogate may speak for a patient ONLY when a
  patient is unable to speak [or write their wishes] on their own behalf):
    List of surrogate decision-maker choices such as health care power of attorney or they have
    not discussed their wishes with the surrogate
  Intubation and Mechanical Ventilation Preferences:
    List of possible wishes for advanced life-prolonging interventions such as intubation or CPR
  Focus of Care:
    Full, selective, or comfort focused
  Resuscitation Preferences:
    Full, DNR-CCA, DNR-CC
  Other Goals of Care Recommendations:
    Narrative of other findings in discussion
    Time spent = *** minutes were spent in the serious illness discussion
    Name of nurse: Date of Service:

Box 4
REMAP a mnemonic to structure serious illness discussions

*R*eframe

*E*xpect emotion

*M*ap out the future

*A*lign with values

*P*lan treatments.

(Vital Talk, 2020)

cancer. Many patients are admitted for symptom management. The critical care nurse works closely with the patient and family during these types of admissions. Many times, it is the critical care nurse who interviews the patient and family on ICU admission and discovers the patient currently using palliative care services. The critical care nurse can inform the health care team of the patient's current palliative care plan and work toward implementation of those pre-ICU interventions that have been successful for the patient. In those instances where the current palliative care plan is not providing relief for the patient, the critical care nurse can work with the inpatient palliative care team to adjust interventions to meet the new patient needs.

Differences in acute care utilization contribute to cost disparities near end of life. One large Medicare study found that medical costs were 32% higher for African Americans than Whites in the last 6 months of life. Approximately 40% of the higher costs were due to greater use of intensive procedures (eg, mechanical ventilation) and admission to the ICU. African Americans are also more likely to die in hospitals compared with Whites, adding to cost differences.[38]

IMPLICATIONS FOR NURSING

Appendix 1 lists identified implications for nursing. A focused literature review tailored to answer questions presented by the case study revealed limited studies exploring the impact of regular serious illness discussions with people of color before admit to the ICU, or to prevent admission to the ICU, or effect on ACP. These authors found no evidence that specifically evaluates interventions that have been effective in decreasing ICU admissions in the African American population with serious life-limiting illnesses. Bedside ICU nurses are invaluable in providing a framework and interventions for further studies.

The establishment of SIC standardized documentation is essential for effective communication between team members. Nurses can identify limitations that prohibit effective documentation of conversations and ease in retrieval of previous conversations to promote productive and therapeutic discussions.

SUMMARY

Prognostic skills have improved dramatically with the advancements in health care. The development of honest, candid, routine conversations with patients with advanced cancer needs to be integrated into their care. This ongoing SIC provides support for patients with advanced cancer as they face their end of life and ideally the time and opportunity to complete any unfinished business and face death on their own terms as much as possible. The health care teams' role is to listen, educate, guide, share the patient's perspective to all team members, and strive to provide goal concordant care. Accessible, practical documentation methods, such as using templates, can expedite communication between team members and provide an excellent method for nurses to provide their unique insights and perspectives to the health care team.

People of color present specific challenges to end-of-life care, particularly in the ICU. Their perspective is impacted by cultural aspects, spiritual beliefs, communication, and trust issues. There is a need for expanded studies to evaluate people of color's perceptions of the ICU and serious life-limiting illnesses. The bedside RN is best positioned to advocate, assess, and participate in conversations related to serious illness.

DISCLOSURE

The authors have nothing to disclose.

APPENDIX: 1: IMPLICATIONS FOR NURSING

- ACP using SICs, framed using the REMAP format, should start early in the cancer illness trajectory and be clearly documented for all the team to review.
- Nurses are an integral part of ACP and contribute invaluable information including patient and family's cultural beliefs. Tripp-Reimer's questions can guide this nursing assessment and drive education.
- Nurses, as patient advocates, can ensure that all patients, including people of color, have the opportunity to express their wishes during SICs.
- Nurses and the remainder of the health care team can use a template to document SICs to increase understanding of the patients' understanding of their disease, care plan, cultural beliefs, and wishes.

REFERENCES

1. Lutz K, Rowniak SR, Sandhu P. A contemporary paradigm: integrating spirituality in advance care planning. J Relig Health 2018;57(2):662–71.
2. Wilkie D, Hoening N, Suarez M, et al. Predicting survival with the palliative performance scale in a minority-serving hospice and palliative care program. J Pain Symptom Manage 2009;37(4):642–8.
3. Gilligan T, Bohlke K, Baile WF. Patient-clinician communication: American Society of clinical Oncology Consensus Guideline summary. J Oncol Pract 2018; 14(1):42–6.
4. Curtis JR, Downey L, Back AL, et al. Effect of a patient and clinician communication-priming intervention on patient-reported goals-of-care discussions between patients with serious illness and clinicians: a randomized clinical trial. JAMA Intern Med 2018;178(7):930–40.
5. Temel JS, Greer JA, Muzikansky A, et al. Early palliative care for patients with metastatic non-small-cell lung cancer. N Engl J Med 2010;363(8):733–42.
6. Smith-Howell E, Hickman S, Meghani S, et al. End-of-Life decision making communication of bereaved family members of African Americans with serious illness. J Palliat Med 2016;19(2):174–82.
7. Mack JW, Cronin A, Taback N, et al. End-of-life care discussions among patients with advanced cancer: a cohort study. Ann Intern Med 2012;156(3):204–10.
8. Emiloju OE, Djibo DAM, Ford JG. Association between the timing of goals-of-care discussion and hospitalization outcomes in patients with metastatic cancer. Am J Hosp Palliat Care 2020;37(6):433–8.
9. Almalki H, Absi A, Alghamdi A, et al. Analysis of patient-physician concordance in the understanding of chemotherapy treatment plans among patients with cancer. JAMA Netw Open 2020;3(3):e200341.
10. Shirado A, Morita T, Akazawa T, et al. Both maintaining hope and preparing for death: effects of physicians' and nurses' behaviors from bereaved family members' perspectives. J Pain Symptom Manage 2013;45(5):848–58.
11. Apostol CC, Waldfogel JM, Pfoh ER, et al. Association of goals of care meetings for hospitalized cancer patients at risk for critical care with patient outcomes. Palliat Med 2015;29(4):386–90.

12. Gieniusz M, Nunes R, Saha V, et al. Earlier goals of care discussions in hospitalized terminally ill patients and the quality of end-of-life care: a Retrospective study. Am J Hosp Palliat Care 2018;35(1):21–7.
13. Hanson LC, Collichio F, Bernard SA, et al. Integrating palliative and Oncology care for patients with advanced cancer: a quality improvement intervention. J Palliat Med 2017;20(12):1366–71.
14. Haun MW, Estel S, Rücker G, et al. Early palliative care for adults with advanced cancer. Cochrane Database Syst Rev 2017;6(6):CD011129.
15. Starr LT, Ulrich CM, Corey KL, et al. Associations among end-of-life discussions, health-care utilization, and costs in persons with advanced cancer: a Systematic review. Am J Hosp Palliat Care 2019;36(10):913–26.
16. Bernacki RE, Block SD. Communication about serious illness care goals: a review and synthesis of best practices. JAMA Intern Med 2014;174(12):1994–2003.
17. Bergqvist J, Strang P. The will to live – breast cancer patients perceptions' of palliative chemotherapy. Acta Oncol 2017;56(9):1168–74.
18. Sudore RL, Lum HD, You JJ, et al. Defining advance care planning for adults: a consensus definition from a multidisciplinary Delphi Panel. J Pain Symptom Manage 2017;53(5):821–32.e1.
19. Pun BT, Balas MC, Barnes-Daly MA, et al. Caring for critically ill patients with the ABCDEF bundle: results of the ICU liberation collaborative in over 15,000 adults. Crit Care Med 2019;47(1):3–14.
20. Weber ML, Byrd C, Cape K, et al. Implementation of the ABDCEF bundle in an Academic medical Center. J Clin Outcomes Manage 2017;24(9).
21. Bernacki R, Hutchings M, Vick J, et al. Development of the Serious Illness Care Program: a randomized controlled trial of a palliative care communication intervention. BMJ Open 2015;5(10):e009032.
22. Sanders J, Robinson M, Block S. Factors impacting advance care planning among African Americans: results of a Systematic integrated review. J Palliat Med 2016;19(2):202–27.
23. Chandar M, Brockstein B, Zunamon A, et al. Perspectives of health-care providers toward advance care planning in patients with advanced cancer and Congestive Heart failure. Am J Hosp Palliat Care 2017;34(5):423–9.
24. You JJ, Downar J, Fowler RA, et al. Barriers to goals of care discussions with seriously ill hospitalized patients and their families: a multicenter survey of clinicians [published correction appears in JAMA Intern Med. 2015 Apr;175(4):659]. JAMA Intern Med 2015;175(4):549–56.
25. Ethier JL, Paramsothy T, You JJ, et al. Perceived barriers to goals of care discussions with patients with advanced cancer and their families in the ambulatory setting: a multicenter survey of oncologists. J Palliat Care 2018;33(3):125–42.
26. Kapo JM, Casarett D. Prognosis in chronic diseases. Ann Long Term Care 2006;14(2).
27. Weng LC, Huang HL, Wiklie DJ, et al. Predicting survival with the palliative performance scale in a minority-serving hospice and palliative care program. J Pain Symptom Manage 2009;37(4):642–8.
28. Address goals of care. Available at: https://www.vitaltalk.org/topics/reset-goals-of-care/. Accessed July 23, 2021.
29. Jonnalagadda S, Lin JJ, Nelson JE, et al. Racial and ethnic differences in beliefs about lung cancer care. Chest 2012;142(5):1251–8.
30. Ejem DB, Barrett N, Rhodes RL, et al. Reducing disparities in the quality of palliative care for older African Americans through improved advance care planning: study Design and Protocol. J Palliat Med 2019;22(S1):90–100.

31. Kemp C. Culture issues in palliative care. Semin Oncol Nurs 2005;21(1):44–52.
32. Tripp-Reimer T, Brink PJ, Saunders JM. Cultural assessment: Content and process. Nurs Outlook 1984;32:78–82.
33. Dillon E, Chuang J, Gupta A, et al. Provider perspectives on advance care planning documentation in the electronic health record: the experience of primary care providers and specialists using advance health-care directives and physician orders for life-sustaining treatment. Am J Hosp Palliat Care 2017;34(10): 918–24.
34. Saiki C, Ferrell B, Longo-Schoeberlein D, et al. Goals-of-care discussions. J Community Support Oncol 2017;15(4):e190–4.
35. Austin CA, Mohottige D, Sudore RL, et al. Tools to promote shared decision making in serious illness: a systematic review. JAMA Intern Med 2015;175(7): 1213–21.
36. Childers JW, Arnold RM. Expanding goals of care conversations across a health system: the mapping the future program. J Pain Symptom Manage 2018;56(4): 637–44.
37. Geerse OP, Lamas DJ, Sanders JJ, et al. A qualitative study of serious illness conversations in patients with advanced cancer. J Palliat Med 2019;22(7): 773–81.
38. Starr LT, Ulrich CM, Appel SM, et al. Goals-of-Care consultations are associated with lower costs and less acute care use among propensity-matched Cohorts of African Americans and whites with serious illness. J Palliat Med 2020;23(9): 1204–13.

New Graduate Nurses in the Intensive Care Setting

Preparing Them for Patient Death

Colette D. Baudoin, PhD (c), MSN, RN, OCN, CNE[a],*,
Aimme Jo McCauley, DNP, MSN, RN[b],
Alison H. Davis, PhD, RN, CNE, CHSE[c]

KEYWORDS

- New graduate nurse • Stress • Intensive care setting • Transition • End-of-life care
- Palliative care • Residency programs

KEY POINTS

- As student nurses transition to practicing nurses, many factors, including the practice readiness gap, lead to burnout and high turnover rates.
- The nursing shortage and recent COVID-19 pandemic has increased the need for new graduate nurses to enter directly into critical care areas upon graduation.
- Intensive care areas complicate the difficult transition process for new graduate nurses with higher acuity patients and increased patient deaths.
- Education regarding end-of-life care and palliative care for new graduate nurses in critical care areas is needed to support new graduate nurse role transition.
- End-of-life and palliative care education provided to new nurse graduates in intensive care areas improves confidence, knowledge, and resilience, while improving patient outcomes.

INTRODUCTION

Nursing is consistently ranked as one of the most stressful professions in health care.[1] Stress and burnout have been researched in nursing since the 1970s as a means to retain nurses and impact the nursing shortage.[1] Nurses consistently identify feelings of being overworked, unable to meet the needs of their patients, inadequately prepared, and unprepared to cope with patient deaths as sources of stress which impact their careers. These sources of stress impact nurses in all stages of their careers,

[a] School of Nursing, Louisiana State University Health Sciences Center New Orleans, 1900 Gravier Street, #417, New Orleans, LA 70112, USA; [b] School of Nursing, Louisiana State University Health Sciences Center New Orleans, 1900 Gravier Street, #5B7, New Orleans, LA 70112, USA; [c] School of Nursing, Louisiana State University Health Sciences Center New Orleans, 1900 Gravier Street, #509, New Orleans, LA 70112, USA
* Corresponding author.
E-mail address: cbaud4@lsuhsc.edu

Crit Care Nurs Clin N Am 34 (2022) 91–101
https://doi.org/10.1016/j.cnc.2021.11.007
ccnursing.theclinics.com

nationally and internationally. New graduate nurses (NGNs) are more vulnerable because of various factors, most notably, the practice readiness gap.

HISTORY AND DEFINITIONS

Historically, the literature describes the transition period from student nurse to registered general nurse or NGN as a stressful time in a nurse's career.[2,3] The initial work experience of a NGN has been described as the sensation of experiencing a reality shock.[4] Reality shock was then defined as "the shock-like reaction that occurs when an individual who has been reared and educated in that subculture of nursing that is promulgated by schools of nursing suddenly discovers that nursing as practiced in the world of work is not the same-it does not operate on the same principles".[5]

The phenomenon of student nurses transitioning to NGNs became more evident during the United States' response to the novel coronavirus disease 2019 (COVID-19) pandemic. As the numbers of COVID-19 cases were increasing rapidly in hospitals throughout the United States in March, April, and May of 2020, many student nurses nearing graduation from nursing school were quickly recruited into intensive care hospital settings as their first job as a NGN.[6] Along with the usual stressors experienced by NGNs, including learning hospital policies and procedures, roles, responsibilities, and complex tasks beyond the nurse generalists role that are required to work in an intensive care setting, the additional stressors of a global pandemic, staffing shortages, lack of personal protective equipment, and a mounting number of critically ill patients, many of whom were infected with the highly contagious COVID-19 virus, required these NGNs to perform their role on the health care team as nurses who had only begun to understand, yet alone master, the complex content and environment of the intensive care setting. Programs are in place to assist NGNs to transition into their roles as nurses, such as new nurse residency programs and/or preceptor programs. During the COVID-19 pandemic, however, preceptors and fellow staff members were struggling themselves to cope with the rapidly changing and uncertain environment.[7]

End-of-life and/or palliative care, especially surrounding communication, is another stressor in the intensive care setting that NGNs must add to their responsibilities in their new, intense work environment. The practice readiness gap is evident here as schools of nursing focus on the care of patients throughout the lifespan, but not the care of the dying patient. Death education should include palliative and end-of-life care. Internationally, there are inconsistencies in death education for undergraduate nurses including "quality, content, and approach."

Many patients in the intensive care settings are nonverbal for numerous reasons and the nurse must try to facilitate family communication and closure at the end of life for these patients in nontraditional methods. Communication is a difficult task alone when patients are ill. With the addition of the intensive care setting and/or the inability to communicate, the end-of-life or palliative care patient has added complex needs and the NGN is now facilitating family communications among themselves and the health care team. Survey results note that 75% of frontline health care workers under the age of 30 years reported a negative impact on their mental health since the beginning of the COVID-19 pandemic with 69% reporting feeling "burned out."[9] With an ever-present and looming nursing shortage, it is important to consider how NGNs can be adequately supported to ensure their success and commitment to continue their goals of working and succeeding in an intensive care setting. The burnout noted surrounding end-of-life and palliative care patients is especially concerning and should be addressed to further ensure the continued success of the NGN in the intensive care setting.

BACKGROUND OF THE NGN

As student nurses graduate from nursing school, they are met with a mix of excitement surrounding graduation and the challenge of preparing to take the National Council Licensure Examination (NCLEX). The multiple stressors and steep learning curves continue as the NGN prepares to apply for and receives their first job as a registered nurse, starts their job, begins a NGN residency program, and begins to develop trusting relationships with a preceptor or preceptors. As a NGN, expectations are to independently implement all assessment and nursing skills and tasks learned as a student while learning the roles and responsibilities of a NGN. NGNs were once encouraged to work on units that would provide a variety of patient care experiences, but with lower patient acuity levels, such as medical-surgical, telemetry, or step-down units.[10] The nationwide nursing shortage, associated with a variety of factors such as the aging workforce, increasing nurse-patient ratios, perceptions of lack of support at work, and reported feelings of job-associated burnout, has led to the need for NGNs to be recruited and hired directly into intensive care settings.[9,10] NGNs do not have the opportunity to experience a variety of patient care experiences at lower acuities, nor experience the care of end of life or palliative care patients, as NGNs are accepting first jobs in the intensive care areas at rates that vary from 18% to 23%.[11]

NGNs are excited to start what is deemed to be an enviable position in the intensive care setting as they did not have to wait to specialize or gain experience in a lower acuity area before entering intensive care. However, the added stressors of learning to care for critically ill patients, in addition to refining nursing assessment skills and procedures, as well as time management and delegation, can be difficult for NGNs.[11] The literature notes the existence of a practice readiness gap between nursing curricula and clinical practice experienced by the NGN hired into the intensive care setting.[11,12] Adding to the complexity of the situation, NCLEX confirms that the NGN has entry-level knowledge; however, intensive care nursing "requires in-depth knowledge of advanced assessment and technologies in managing life-threatening, complex nursing situations."[11]

An added complexity to this already intense work environment, the NGN is often tasked with managing patients and families that require not just intense physical care, but psychological and emotional care and counsel as they transition to end-of-life or palliative care. The patient requiring this specialized care may or may not be able to communicate fully, adding another layer of stress and complexity to their care. This complexity results in the NGN reporting a higher amount of work-related stress than their experienced nurse counterparts in the intensive care setting.[13] As colleagues, nurse educators, and employers of NGN, they must receive the support and assistance necessary to facilitate the transition from the role of a nursing student to a NGN working in the intensive care environment where patient acuity is high, technology is complex, and the saving lives is the focus. In the intensive care setting, the reality is that not every life can be saved and/or some patients have reached the end of their lives. An understanding and knowledge of palliative and end-of-life care is needed in the intensive care setting to assist NGN to transition to their roles and decrease the reported feelings of job burnout while decreasing the practice readiness gap and turnover rates.[11,12]

The turnover rate for nurses in the acute care setting averaged 19.5% in 2020 with NGN turnover reported to be as high as 23.9% and 17% in the intensive care setting.[11,14] Literature reports that new nurses lack confidence and report feeling uncomfortable when starting their new nursing positions.[11,12] It should be noted that NGNs will not begin to feel confident until at least year 2 of their practice. This phenomenon can be explained based on Benner's novice to expert continuum and novice nurses (ie, new nurses) "tend to exhibit competence toward the end of the second year of practice."[11] Competence can lead to confidence as the NGN begins to believe they can handle the stressors of the intensive care environment. The impact of the theory-practice gap has been explored for NGNs in the critical care environment. Findings indicate that knowledge and skill acquisition, workplace culture, and having a resource person are essential for the NGN to transition successfully into the intensive care setting.[15] There is no additional training required to enter practice into the intensive care setting for NGNs, even though the expectations and high acuity of patients are well known. The high-level practice expectations in the intensive care setting result in emotional stress for new nurses.[11,13]

Providing nursing care for a patient at their end of life in an intensive care setting can be problematic for even experienced nurses.[16] End-of-life and palliative care has become a recognized component of the intensive care nurse's role, whether experienced or new, and the nurse must be comfortable with this role and its responsibilities.[16] In the intensive care setting, death can be a common occurrence with death rates ranging from 10% to 29%.[17]

Communication skills are key for the NGN when a patient is at the end of life and actively dying, but they may not have received this training in nursing school.[8] Collaboration with the interprofessional team and communication with families can be "especially stressful for nurses."[16] NGNs find themselves caring not only for the dying patient, but also for the family as other members of the health care team leave for other responsibilities. Emotional and psychological distress and burden can result from attempts to provide care to the patient and family simultaneously, which NGNs have not been specifically trained to do.[8,16,18] Owing to their inexperience, NGNs may face ethical and moral dilemmas as they struggle with feelings that the intensive care setting may not be an ideal place for end-of-life care.[19,20] There is a noted gap in the literature as little evidence is available addressing the support and skills needed for the NGN to care and manage the critical care patient competently, confidently, and empathetically at end of life.

Support for the NGN

A solution to address the turnover rate and other issues that NGNs face, such as the practice readiness gap, was the development of nurse residency programs. Nurse residency programs were designed to support the professional growth of NGNs and support their transition to independent nurses.[21] Nurse residency programs vary in format and content, but the 3 most common programs in place are didactic-based, simulation-based, and clinical preceptorship-based.[22] Nurse residency programs can incorporate orientation programs of other organizations such as the Association of Critical Care Nursing or Association of Women's Health, Obstetric, and Neonatal Nurses. Nurse residency programs vary from 10 to 15 months in length and content can include critical thinking skills, clinical decision making, communication, professional growth through preceptorship experiences, and assimilating to the role of the nurse.[21] Outcomes of nurse residency programs have been noted as positive and include increased retention, improvements in job satisfaction within the first year, and improvements to clinical decision-making.[22] Nurse residency programs do not include care for the end-of-life patient nor palliative care and is a noted gap in the literature. Inclusion of end-of-life care and palliative care content that would assist NGNs to transition into the intensive care setting and could impact the experience of reality shock.[4]

DISCUSSION

Nurse residency programs are designed and developed to meet the needs of the organization in assuring that NGNs can meet the needs of the patients they care for on a regular basis.[22] Unfortunately, these programs often overlook the practice readiness gap and/or knowledge gap from the undergraduate curricula that NGNs have in managing the patient at the end of life who may have additional complex care needs such as emotional needs or communication requirements with family concerning their status.[8] The knowledge required to meet the needs of an intensive care patient is undisputable, and despite advances in science and medicine, death in the intensive care setting is common. Therefore, it is essential for NGNs to receive adequate preparation to manage the end-of-life patient to be successful beyond the first year of hire in the intensive care setting.

The Association of Critical Care Nursing's (ACCN) orientation program, Essentials of Critical Care Orientation (ECCO), includes more than 75 continuing education (CE) credits for participants, yet only one part of one module totaling 4.4 CEs addresses the mechanics of managing a palliative care patient. This calculates to 5.9% of the total ECCO curriculum as dedicated to palliative care. There is a need for specific knowledge, tasks, and nursing care on end-of-life and palliative care to be addressed for NGNs, yet there remains a lack of resources and evidence-based literature. There is a paucity of literature addressing the role transition of NGNs through either a nurse residency program or a new nurse orientation program that includes the nursing care of the end-of-life patient.[23,24] Specifically, the physical, emotional, or psychological care of the end-of-life patient should be included in the content for NGNs for successful retention in the intensive care area beyond 1 year.[11,12] If this gap remains, NGNs will continue to experience inadequate role transition as well as experience the inability to develop the necessary communication skills, empathetic management, and grit to care for the end-of-life or palliative care intensive care patient and the circle of insecurities and anxieties often reported by NGNs will continue to perpetuate in this population of nurses.

Clinical Relevance

The cost of orienting a NGN is reported to be more expensive than an experienced nurse at a staggering range of $60,000 to $96,000.[22] Estimates show that it takes approximately 137 nonproductive hours to fully orient a new nurse.[25] Once orientation is complete, NGN retention is imperative and nurse residency programs have shown to decrease turnover rates by 36%.[22] The cost to an organization to replace a nurse's position is reported to be approximately one-half of that nurse's salary.[10]

More than cost-savings to the organization though is the positive patient outcomes for the patients cared for and the overall health and well-being of the nurses caring for them. Optimum end-of-life care for patients and families has the ability to provide a lasting memory for the family members that can be carried forward. The feelings from the experience brought forward by the nurse caring for that patient and family can also leave a lasting imprint on the career of that nurse. Intensive care nurses caring for patients at the end of life reported that "critical care nurses need more knowledge, skill, and sense of cultural competency to provide quality care"[26] to patients being cared for at end of life in order to be assured that the care is meaningful and appropriate for the given situation. The nurses felt they were lacking knowledge in pain management, symptom management, ethical issues, and communication with families and care during the last hours of life that needed to be provided.[26] These needs were gathered from a population of nurses with an average of 11 years of intensive care experience, although 39% of respondents had less than 4 years of experience. If experienced nurses are struggling with these issues, then the added stress of being a NGN in the intensive care setting has the potential to amplify these needs to care for patients at the end of life. To promote resilience in these NGNs, it is essential to promote teamwork, mentoring, and exposure to varying situations.[11] This includes situations surrounding management of patients at the end of life.

FUTURE DIRECTIONS
Palliative-Specific Support for New Nurses

The NGN enters the intensive care setting with the intention of providing curative care and treatments to patients with life-threatening illnesses.[16,26] Forming perceptions of critically ill patients, care, and outcomes based on didactic and clinical experiences in undergraduate education, the new nurse is not prepared to manage the realities of death and end-of-life or palliative care in the intensive care area.[8,27] Traditional hospital onboarding, orientation, nurse residency programs, and professional developmental support programs lack educational content and experiences to support new nurses in caring for dying patients and their families. Focused education and experiences in palliative care and supportive environments are required to achieve the high-quality end-of-life care.[28]

NGNs report feeling unprepared, unsupported, inexperienced, and emotional distress and isolation after a first-time patient death.[16,19] Historically, intensive care nurses have coped with psychological impacts, including depression, moral distress, secondary trauma, performance guilt, and eventual burnout related to experiences in palliative and end-of-life care because of a lack of supplemental education and psychological support.[29] To gain the necessary skills to provide end-of-life or palliative care, NGNs require education specific to end-of-life or palliative care goals and the physiology of death, a supportive environment providing experiential learning during nurse residency programs, written policies, and interprofessional agreements pertaining to end-of-life care, structured debriefing after patient death encounters in the residency period and in postresidency practice, and resilience education that provides tools and practices to sustain mental health and well-being after end-of-life or palliative experiences.[27]

Palliative Education

The prerequisite for quality end-of-life care is comprehensive palliative care education and competency. Although undergraduate nursing programs do include education on hospice, palliative care, and end-of-life care, the didactic content is inconsistent and rarely translated to practicum education, as most end-of-life experiences have limited clinical opportunities for students because of the sensitivity required for patients and their families.[28,30,31] Incorporating the End-of-Life Nursing Education Consortium [ELNEC] Project's Undergraduate Curriculum into NGN residency and/or orientation programs, dependent on the institution, provides end-of-life and palliative specific education, which can be purposefully implemented in the intensive care environment. The ELNEC curriculum comprises the following 6 modules: an introduction to the nurse's role in palliative care, enhanced communication techniques, pain management goals and ethical considerations, symptom management for dying patients, coping and support strategies for nurses and families of dying patients, and the management of the physiologic, cultural, spiritual, and social dimensions surrounding death.[30] NGNs who received ELNEC education during nurse residency programs reported being able to apply specific interventions and knowledge to their first end-of-life experience. These NGNs reported statistically significant increases (p = .001) in 7 of 8 survey questions using a 10-point Likert scale, to include comfort ($M = 7.7$), competence ($M = 7.7$), and knowledge in providing palliative care ($M = 8.2$), pain assessment and management ($M = 8.4$), symptom assessment or management ($M = 8.1$), communication in serious illness ($M = 7.5$), loss grief bereavement ($M = 7.2$), and caring for a patient in final hours ($M = 7.1$).[30]

Enhanced communication skills needed to manage palliative care requires specialized training for the NGN.[28,30,32] As attention shifts from the dying patient to the family during death, NGNs are often overwhelmed by family needs, questions, and emotions; all while coping with their own personal beliefs, awareness of, and inexperience with death.[17,32] Lacking confidence, experience, and knowledge, the NGN may avoid the patient and family, and use vague and evasive communication techniques because of inexperience and lack of confidence.[17] Simulation for palliative and end-of-life care events can provide NGNs with a safe and controlled experience for practicing therapeutic communication with dying patients and families, model professional behaviors and dialogue in palliative care, and reduce event-related feelings of being overwhelmed by providing early opportunities for self-reflection and insight into the NGN's own beliefs about death and loss through reflection and debriefing. Simulation standards of best practice close all simulation events with debriefing, another opportunity for reflection and closure of the experience.[33]

The NGN has novice level experience in the assessment, ethical and safety considerations, and pain management of patients with transient illness, with the expectation that pain will gradually lessen with healing and eventually resolve, correlating with the goal of reducing pain medication. NGNs report avoidance, frustration, and moral distress during end-of-life care, with the fear of hastening death.[27,30,34] Having limited to no palliative practicum experiences, new nurses lack the knowledge, confidence, and skills to pharmaceutically facilitate palliative goals.[27,31] Pain management education for the end-of-life and/or palliative patient informs NGNs that end-of-life pain management goals cannot be accomplished solely with foundational pain management skills, and requires understanding that palliative pain management addresses many symptoms other than pain, specific interventions for obtaining comfort through stages of dying, and that the pathophysiological knowledge of death for the education and support families of dying patients through this process is essential.[27,28,32]

The greatest challenges in palliative nursing care are the shifting of care goals from patient to the family and managing the internal and external stressors of death and dying. This shifting of priorities of care requires specialized training, self-reflection, peer support, and opportunities for integration for the NGN. Education, including grief, loss, the physiology of death, honoring cultural needs and unique family requests, and how to manage, support, and respect the family and wishes of dying clients, provides NGNs the ability to fully engage as the coordinator of care.[27,28,30,32]

Supportive Environment

Numerous effective and evidenced-based programs for peer and environmental support are available to provide NGNs with experience and the necessary support in end-of-life and palliative care. Transitional support programs, such as preceptorship, peer coaching, mentorship, and nurse residency programs, which include direct and intentional exposure to palliative and end-of-life experiences with experienced nurses, provide the necessary exposure, wisdom, and opportunity to observe professional, proficient nursing management of dying patients and their families.[11,21,26,27,31] Death is not unique to the intensive care environment.[17] Nurses, especially NGNs, must be able to recognize when additional support is needed, whether for themselves and/ or for coworkers. Without the engagement of peer support systems, the NGN can experience emotional isolation, distress, and powerlessness, resulting in low-quality palliative outcomes, burnout, and depression.[17,28]

Palliative Policies and Agreements

Institutional policies on palliative care and end-of-life procedures provide concrete guidelines and references, underpin interprofessional agreements and shared expectations, support appropriate decision-making, and reduce barriers and stressors for nurses providing end-of-life and palliative care.[26–28,32] Hospitals and organizations should provide documented policies, procedures, and resources for end-of-life and palliative care that are reliable and administratively supported for NGNs to review and confidently use when sharing information with families, honoring family requests, or managing interprofessional disagreements. Instituting palliative and end-of-life policies and procedures increases patient care quality and outcomes, and reduces feelings of NGN powerlessness, stress, confusion, and conflict, allowing NGNs to build confidence and decision-making abilities surrounding this stressful topic.[27,28,32]

Debriefing

Evidence-based simulation and education in end-of-life and palliative care introduces the NGN to structured debriefing methods. Structured debriefing after the end-of-life or palliative care is an evidence-based method for preventing unresolved emotional and psychological impacts of moral and emotional distress and secondary trauma.[16,27,33,34] Debriefing should consistently be used by health care teams after all death events to support emotional well-being, improvements in future care and practice, and provide event closure for all health care providers.[29,33,34] Debriefing is especially important for the NGN, as internal beliefs and context surrounding death and dying are likely only in the formative stages.[16,27,33] NGNs need the support that debriefing can provide through the facilitation of self-reflection, peer-to-peer sharing, discussion of ethical issues and concepts in palliative decision-making, and opportunities for improvement in nursing practice.[16,27,33–35]

Resilience Training

Resilience training provides education and opportunities supporting NGNs in managing the psychological, physiologic, emotional, and spiritual impacts caused by stress and high-stress events, such as the death of a patient or conflict with the family of a dying patient. Psychological impacts encountered include guilt, bereavement, moral distress, emotional distress, and secondary trauma, which can significantly impact the quality of care and the well-being of the NGN, and indirectly impact the palliative outcomes of the dying patient.[11,17,27,29,34] Throughout palliative programs, education, and sustained support systems for NGNs, consistent and frequent promotion of self-care, self-assessments for well-being, and tools for resilience are evidenced to positively impact empowerment, work satisfaction, critical thinking, competency, and the quality of care delivered.[11,17,27,29,34]

SUMMARY

The transition period for NGNs is historically a time of increased stress. NGNs are known to experience a practice readiness gap, especially in the areas of palliative care and end-of-life care. Undergraduate nursing curricula are inconsistent in the provision of content on death and dying, further compounding the problem. Nurse residency programs have the opportunity to offer this much-needed education to NGNs. With the inclusion of palliative and end-of-life care content, nurse residency programs can reduce stress, burnout, and turnover rates in NGNs while impacting the quality of patient care for the dying patient and their families. The circle of life includes death and so the topics of palliative and end-of-life care must be addressed so that patients and their families can benefit from an increased quality of care provided by a confident, satisfied, resilient nurse, no matter the stage of their career.

CLINICS CARE POINTS

- In the intensive care setting, new graduate nurses report higher work-related stress and will not begin to feel confident until at least year 2 of their practice
- Nurse residency programs support the professional growth of new graduate nurses and decrease turnover rates by 36%
- New graduate nurses need palliative and end-of-life education to supplement the readiness to practice gap
- Nurse residency programs should include palliative and end-of-life care content as well as mentoring and simulation to guide and support professional development and exploration of internal beliefs and content surrounding death and dying
- Positive patient and family outcomes can result from new graduate nurses who attend nurse residency programs with palliative and end-of-life care content

DISCLOSURE

The authors have nothing to disclose.

REFERENCES

1. Redfearn RA, van Ittersum KW, Stenmark CK. The impact of sensory processing sensitivity on stress and burnout in nurses. Int J Stress Manag 2020;27(4):370–9.
2. Godinez G, Schweiger J, Gruver J, et al. Role transition from graduate to staff nurse: a qualitative analysis. J Nurses Staff Dev 1999;15(3):97–110.
3. O'kane CE. Newly qualified nurses experiences in the intensive care unit. Nurs Crit Care 2012;17(1):44–51.
4. Kramer. Reality shock: why nurses leave nursing: AJN the American Journal of Nursing. The American Journal of Nursing; 1974. Available at: https://journals.lww.com/ajnonline/Citation/1975/05000/REALITY_SHOCK__Why_Nurses_Leave_Nursing.41.aspx. [Accessed 1 August 2021].
5. Kramer: Current issues in nursing - Google Scholar. Available at: https://scholar.google.com/scholar_lookup?title=Current+Issues+in+Nursing&author=M+Kramer&publication_year=1985&. [Accessed 1 August 2021].
6. A timeline of COVID-19 developments in 2020. Available at: https://www.ajmc.com/view/a-timeline-of-covid19-developments-in-2020. [Accessed 1 August 2021].
7. Arnetz JE, Goetz CM, Arnetz BB, et al. Nurse reports of stressful situations during the COVID-19 pandemic: qualitative analysis of survey responses. Int J Environ Res Public Health 2020;17(21):8126.

8. Cavaye J, Watts JH, Mcilfatrick S, et al. An integrated literature review of death education in pre-registration nursing curricula: key themes. Int J Palliat Care 2014;2014:1–19.

9. Kirzinger A, Kearney A, Hamel L, et al. KFF/Washington Post Frontline Health Care Workers Survey – Vaccine Intentions – 9666 | KFF. Kaiser Fam Found. 2021. Available at: https://www.kff.org/report-section/kff-washington-post-frontline-health-care-workers-survey-vaccine-intentions/ [Accessed 31 July 2021].

10. Steele-Moses S, Creel E, Carruth A. Recruitment attributes important to new nurse graduates employed on adult medical-surgical units. Medsurg Nurs 2018;27(5):310–28.

11. DeGrande H, Liu F, Greene P, et al. The experiences of new graduate nurses hired and retained in adult intensive care units. Intensive Crit Care Nurs 2018; 49:72–8.

12. Casey K, Tsai CL, Fink RM. A psychometric evaluation of the casey-fink graduate nurse experience survey. J Nurs Adm 2021;51(5):242–8.

13. Feddeh SA, Darawad MW. Correlates to work-related stress of newly-graduated nurses in critical care units. Int J Caring Sci 2020;13(1):507–16.

14. 2021 NSI National Health Care Retention & RN Staffing report. Available at: www.nsinursingsolutions.com. [Accessed 31 July 2021].

15. Cunnington T, Calleja P. Transition support for new graduate and novice nurses in critical care settings: an integrative review of the literature. Nurse Educ Pract 2018;30(January):62–72.

16. Jang SK, Park WH, Kim HI, et al. Exploring nurses' end-of-life care for dying patients in the ICU using focus group interviews. Intensive Crit Care Nurs 2019; 52:3–8.

17. Rivera-Romero N, Ospina Garzón HP, Henao-Castaño AM. The experience of the nurse caring for families of patients at the end of life in the intensive care unit. Scand J Caring Sci 2019;33(3):706–11.

18. Vanderspank-Wright B, Fothergill-Bourbonnais F, Malone-Tucker S, et al. Nurse graduates' perceived educational needs after the death of a patient: a descriptive qualitative research study. J Contin Educ Nurs 2018;33(3):267–73.

19. Mani ZA. Intensive care unit nurses experirnces of providing end of life care. Middle East J Nurs 2016;10(1):3–9.

20. Sullivan DR, Curtis JR. A view from the frontline: palliative and ethical considerations of the COVID-19 pandemic. J Palliat Med 2021;24(2):293–5.

21. Casey K, Fink R, Krugman M, et al. The graduate nurse experience. J Nurs Adm 2004;34(6):303–11.

22. Perron T, Gascoyne M, Kallakavumkal TK, et al. Effectiveness of nurse residency programs. J Nurs Pract Appl Rev Res 2009;9(2):48–53.

23. Short K, Freedman K, Matays J, et al. Making the transition: a critical care skills program to support newly hired nurses. Clin Nurse Spec 2019;33(3):123–7.

24. Bortolotto SJ. Developing a comprehensive critical care orientation program for graduate nurses. J Nurses Prof Dev 2015;31(4):203–10.

25. Herleth A, Virkstis K, Renfroe J, et al. The challenging road to clinical competence for new graduate RNs. J Nurs Adm 2020;50(4):185–6.

26. Crump SK, Schaffer MA, Schulte E. Critical care nurses' perceptions of obstacles, supports, and knowledge needed in providing quality end-of-life care. Dimens Crit Care Nurs 2010;29(6):297–306.

27. Cadavero AA, Sharts-Hopko NC, Granger BB. Nurse graduates' perceived educational needs after the death of a patient: a descriptive qualitative research study. J Contin Educ Nurs 2020;51(6):267–73.
28. Fridh I. Caring for the dying patient in the ICU - the past, the present and the future. Intensive Crit Care Nurs 2014;30(6):306–11.
29. Badger JM. Critical care nurse intern program. Crit Care Nurs Q 2008;31(2): 184–7.
30. Mazanec P, Ferrell B, Virani R, et al. Preparing new graduate RNs to provide primary palliative care. J Contin Educ Nurs 2020;51(6):280–6.
31. Usher BM, DiNella J, Ren D, et al. Development of end-of-life peer nurse coaches: a hospital-based quality improvement project. J Hosp Palliat Nurs 2015;17(6):551–8.
32. Ganz FDK. Improving family intensive care unit experiences at the end of life: barriers and facilitators. Crit Care Nurse 2019;39(3):52–8.
33. Randall D, Garbutt D, Barnard M. Using simulation as a learning experience in clinical teams to learn about palliative and end-of-life care: a literature review. Death Stud 2018;42(3):172–83.
34. Anniello L, Karl C. Stress debriefing: making the ICU safe for new nurses. Nurs Made Incred Easy! 2021;19(3):22–6.
35. Palmryd L, Rejnö Å, Godskesen TE. Integrity at end of life in the intensive care unit: a qualitative study of nurses' views. Ann Intensive Care 2021;11(1):23.

Perinatal Palliative Care in the Neonatal Intensive Care Unit

Cathy Maher-Griffiths, DNS, MSHCM, RN, RNC-OB, NEA-BC*

KEYWORDS

- Perinatal palliative care • Neonatal palliative care • Resilience • Memory making

KEY POINTS

- With an excess of 20,000 infant deaths occurring in the United States primarily due to congenital malformations and prematurity, many of those infants are receiving perinatal palliative care and are cared for by neonatal intensive care unit (NICU) nurses.
- Providing perinatal palliative care in the NICU requires that NICU nurses have palliative care education and training and resilience building interventions.
- The NICU nurse facilitates memory-making activities that provide significant meaning to the families of infants receiving perinatal palliative care.
- More research on perinatal care processes is an imperative in improving outcomes of care for these infants.

INTRODUCTION

With the frequency of infant deaths and the improvements in prenatal testing, perinatal palliative care (PPC) has become an increasingly important component of neonatal intensive care unit (NICU) care.[1,2] In 2018, there were 21,498 infant deaths reported in the United States, with 27% attributed to congenital malformations and another 17% due to short gestation and low birth weight, and ultimately those babies may require care in the NICU (National Vital Statistics Reports). PPC may be initiated as early as the second trimester of pregnancy, requiring obstetric, maternal-fetal medicine, and neonatal caregiver collaboration (British Association of Perinatal Medicine). Nonetheless, when an infant requiring PPC is admitted to the NICU, the NICU nurse provides clinical care to the infant and extensive supportive care to the family.[3]

Few parents envision that their infants will begin their lives in a NICU, and almost no parent believes at the outset of pregnancy that they will need to discuss the need for PPC.[4] Caring for these infants and their families is difficult and can lead to the NICU nurse experiencing compassion fatigue and burnout.[5] This review describes the

Graduate Program, Louisiana State University Health School of Nursing, New Orleans, LA, USA
* 224 West Greens Drive, Baton Rouge, LA 70810.
E-mail address: mmahe4@lsuhsc.edu

Crit Care Nurs Clin N Am 34 (2022) 103–119
https://doi.org/10.1016/j.cnc.2021.11.008
0899-5885/22/© 2022 Elsevier Inc. All rights reserved.

ccnursing.theclinics.com

essential role of the NICU nurse in the PPC process, the personal impact of providing care to this fragile patient population and their families, and the infrastructure required to deliver PPC effectively. With genomic testing advancing, the use of PPC only will increase.[6] Additionally, although the literature describes neonatal palliative care as a seperate specialty, this review acknowledges the comprehensive approach of PPC, which includes neonatal palliative care.

BACKGROUND

The development of PPC for infants and families has occurred over the past few decades.[1(p35),7,8] From the initial model of perinatal hospice delivering minimal supportive interventions to infants while providing psychosocial support to the families, PPC evolved to providing comprehensive care to infants and families.[1(p35)] Meanwhile, and seemingly concurrently, the PPC movement progressed to include the care of infants with severe anomalies, infants born prior to viability, and infants with overwhelming disease states unresponsive to treatment.[9] Many of these infants and families ultimately are cared for by NICU nurses.

In 2010, candidate conditions for PPC were further defined into 1 of 5 categories: (1) category 1: an antenatal or postnatal diagnoses not compatible with long-term survival; (2) category 2: an antenatal or postnatal condition, which is associated with substantial morbidity or death; (3) category 3: infants born at the margins of viability and for whom intensive care was deemed unsuitable; (4) category 4: postnatal condition with a high risk of severe impairment for the infant's quality of life; and (5) category 5: postnatal conditions that result in the infant having unendurable suffering.[10] When mothers are offered PPC after finding out their infant is in category 1 or category 2, many opt to continue to their pregnancy rather than abort.[11,12]

PPC still is developing as a science and requires undergraduate, postgraduate, and continuing education.[13] Undergraduate and postgraduate PPC education has not been consistently adopted.[13] When an infant is receiving palliative care, NICU nurses must have excellent communication skills when speaking with vulnerable and overwhelmed parents.[4] To that end, PPC presents ethical challenges for the NICU nurse, which can lead to moral distress.[14] NICU nurses have identified the barriers to effective PPC as (1) education, (2) lack of privacy, (3) isolation, (4) staff grief and loss, and (5) policy and procedures.[15]

There is a lack of formalized preparatory education for physicians and nurses who care for infants in the NICU, causing a delay in initiating PPC, leading to lost opportunities for building relationships with the parents, appropriate goal setting, and care of the infant.[16] In 2018, the National Consensus Project for Quality Palliative Care produced the fourth edition of *Clinical Practice Guidelines for Quality Palliative Care*, defining 8 domains of care (**Table 1**).[17]

DEFINING PERINATAL PALLIATIVE CARE

Together for Short Lives (2017) states, "Palliative care for babies, children and young people with life-limiting conditions is an active and total approach to care, from the point of diagnosis or recognition, throughout the child's life and death. It embraces physical, emotional, social and spiritual elements and focuses on the enhancement of the quality of life for the child/young person and support for the family. It includes the management of distressing symptoms, provision of short breaks and care through death and bereavement." "Beneficial at any stage of a serious illness, palliative care is an interdisciplinary care delivery system designated to anticipate, prevent and manage physical, psychological, social and spiritual suffering to optimize the quality

Table 1
Palliative care clinical practice guidelines

Domain	Processes and Aspects of Care	Exemplar
1	Structure	A large hospital system has inpatient palliative care for 15 y. The hospital leadership commits to the growth of perinatal palliative care and assuring that there are hospice programs for neonates.
2	Physical	The pharmacist works with the neonatology team to improve symptom management protocols for infants receiving palliative care.
3	Psychological and psychiatric	In the NICU, the palliative care team collaborates with child life specialists and pediatric clinical psychologists to address the anxiety of the siblings of infants receiving palliative care.
4	Social	A social worker in a community hospice has recognized the need for improving perinatal palliative care. She is empowered by her leadership to reach out to obstetric to co-creating a perinatal palliative care program so that all infants and families receive the appropriate support.
5	Spiritual, religious, and existential	A large health system commits to hiring a board-certified professional chaplain to serve as the leader for the perinatal palliative care coordination. This professional implements a screening tool for spiritual distress.
6	Cultural	The PPC team recognizes the diverse patient population served. Prior to the care meetings, the team meets with the interpreter to prepare for the meeting.
7	Care of the patient nearing the end of life	The neonatal nurse practitioner is certified in palliative care. She collaborates with home health and home hospice to improve end of life care of infants being cared for at home.
8	Ethical and legal	The NICU nurses were experiencing moral distress due to ethical and legal implications of withdrawing life-sustaining measures. A multidisciplinary group, including members from the ethics committee, was convened to standardize the withdrawal of life sustaining measures, including the development of a checklist.

Adapted from Brandt K. Clinical Practice Guidelines for Quality Palliative Care. National Consensus Project for Quality Palliative Care. Available at: https://www.nationalcoalitionhpc.org/wp-content/uploads/2020/07/NCHPC-NCPGuidelines_4thED_web_FINAL.pdf. Accessed June 22, 2021.

of life for patients, their families, and caregivers. Palliative care can be delivered in any care setting through the collaboration of many types of care providers" (National Consensus Project for Quality Palliative Care).[17] PPC is a coordinated method of care for both mother and infant that focuses on maximizing the quality of life and the comfort of infants while supporting the mother and family in pregnancy and beyond (American College of Obstetricians and Gynecologists [ACOG] #786).

In 2020, the World Health Organization[18] defined palliative care: "Palliative care is an approach that improves the quality of life of patients (adults and children) and their families who are facing problems associated with life-threatening illness. It prevents and relieves suffering through the early identification, correct assessment and treatment of pain and other problems, whether physical, psychosocial or spiritual."

An interdisciplinary team approach is required to deliver PPC to the infant and family and initially can include both cure-oriented care and disease-altering care and then shift to exclusively palliative care when that care no longer is effective.[19] PPC is comprehensive and holistic care for parents who are expecting an infant with a life-limiting condition.[20] PPC can be provided to infants for hours, days, weeks, months, or years.[3]

COMPONENTS OF PERINATAL PALLIATIVE CARE PROGRAM

Components of PPC include formal prenatal consultation; development of a birth plan; access to other neonatal and pediatric subspecialties; support and care during the prenatal, birth, and postnatal periods; memory making; and bereavement counseling (ACOG). The NICU should participate in the palliative care consult process, high-risk obstetrics-gynecology multidisciplinary team meetings, and the grief and bereavement plan meetings.[21–23]

Perinatal Palliative Care Consults

With improved technology, infants more frequently are identified who have life-limiting conditions that require the limitation of some treatments and/or withdrawal of treatments in favor of a palliative care approach.[23] Before care planning can commence, parents need complete information and may require multiples session to accomplish this, especially if other pediatric subspecialty consultations are required.

Parents require information that is clear and accurate and that is presented in an empathetic manner, and they need

- The information about what is wrong with the baby explained in simple terms
- The opportunity to discuss how the infant's condition may have an impact on the current pregnancy and how the management of this pregnancy may have an impact on future reproductive health, including the opportunity to have a live birth
- To be told how long their infant may survive and the benefits and risks of available treatments
- To know the possible outcomes if treatments are continued and the effects on their infant
- The likely outcome of a palliative care approach and supports and options available
- To be a major part of the decision-making process
- According to the Victorian Agency for Health Information.[23]

Other information and discussion with parents need to include

- Even though predicting how long the infant will live is difficult, descriptions of how the infant may die
- The idea of living with uncertainty
- Description of what the baby will look like and physical changes as the infant's condition deteriorates, such as coloring and gasping respirations (Victorian Agency for Health Information)

The initial consultation should include the array of decisions that the mother and family may face when the infant is born (ACOG #786). As soon as an infant is named, the PPC team refers to the infant by the given name (ACOG). Other goals of the initial consultation visit are to forge a partnership for ongoing care, to authenticate the mother's decision to pursue palliative care for the infant, and to ensure that the goals are reasonable for the pregnancy (ACOG). For the NICU nurse, spending time as a family usually is a goal that is facilitated in the NICU. Developing a process for mandatory consults for certain diagnoses also improves access to PPC.[24]

Care Planning

The birth plan that is co-created with the family and the interdisciplinary care team includes the prenatal, perinatal, and neonatal periods.[1,25,26] The birth plan is a living document that evolves over time as the condition of the infant changes during the pregnancy, birth, and stay in the NICU.[1] Contingency planning is an important component of the birth plan to account for those changes.[1] The PPC team needs to be mindful that the perception of the quality of life may differ for the parents and the care team.[26]

The PPC plan should include care expectations and wishes for (1) pregnancy, (2) admission to the birthing facility, (3) labor, (4) birth, and (5) neonatal care.[1] The documentation must include these elements:

- PPC team members
- Current list of family's wishes and expectations
- Infant's diagnosis and diagnostic processes
- Comprehensive discussion of initial meetings with family
- Ethics consult results when performed
- Birth planning discussions
- Additional notes and consults[1]

The care planning process provides a full story and provides the family with important documentation of the infant's legacy.[1] This comprehensive care plan provides a road map for the staff, in particular the NICU nurse, to provide care according to the family's wishes.[1,27,28] This document needs to be readily available for the NICU nurses to be able to provide the care that protects, nurtures, and socializes and for designing the care for the infant receiving PPC. This comprehensive care plan, as described by the National Association of Neonatal Nurses (**Fig. 1**).[27]

For babies in categories 1 and 2, PPC is initiated only after a diagnosis has been confirmed and an interdisciplinary team has scrutinized the findings and agree on the diagnosis and prognosis.[10] Once confirmation is made, the parents are notified of the findings and the infants may be candidates for PPC. The initial meeting with the parents may not include all members of the PPC interdisciplinary team; however, ongoing PPC care planning meetings should include, but are not limited to, an obstetrician, neonatologist, NICU nurse, labor and delivery nurse, social worker, and any other relevant pediatric subspecialists.[10]

Additional considerations for the infant's PPC plan should address

- The birth, care, and death of the infant
- Whom they would like present at the infant's birth
- Any ceremony or rituals that are important to the family (naming or baptism)
- Where would they like their infant to die (hospital vs home) (Victorian Agency for Health Information)[23]

The NICU nurse assists with the birth plan for assessment and care of the infant, including bonding, skin-to-skin contact, warmth, hydration, feeding, and lactation (ACOG). It is preferable that the NICU nurse who was part of the palliative care team be present for delivery (ACOG).

Care Delivery

Once an infant has been born and is admitted to the NICU, the care is considered neonatal palliative care, a continuation of PPC, or is distinct should the infant's condition not be identified for palliative care until after birth.[3] Even for infants with PPC

Woman's

■ *Perinatal Palliative Care Plan*

Date of Interview_____

EDC_____

INFANT NAME:_____ACCT #:_____

This perinatal hospice care plan represents my/our wishes for labor, delivery, postpartum care and neonatal care for our baby. I/We have developed this plan with the assistance of Woman's Hospital Social Services Department, Maternal Fetal Medicine physician and neonatology. I/We know that circumstances beyond everyone's control may prevent or change some of the things outlined below, but I/we hope this will serve as a guide for our wishes. I/We understand that our feelings may change and I/we may make adjustments to this care plan as I/we deem necessary throughout this process.

Introduction:

Our baby has been prenatally diagnosed with a life threatening condition.

The prenatal ultrasound revealed _____

We had amniocentesis during pregnancy   ☐ Yes   ☐ No

If yes, amniocentesis showed _____

Labor and Delivery

- I/We have been informed that there is / is not a high risk for stillborn.

- I/We want / do not want our baby's heartbeat to be monitored during labor.

- If there is a loss of heartbeat prior to delivery, I/we do / do not wish to be informed.

  Preferences for pain management and medications include:

  _____

  _____

I/We are aware that there are greater risks to the mother associated with a C-Section delivery when compared to vaginal delivery. I/We know that a C-section may be necessary if an unexpected obstetrical issue arises that puts _____ health in danger. I/We know that a C-section is not a guarantee of a live birth.

- I/We want / do not want a C-section for fetal distress.

- I/We would like _____ to cut the cord after delivery if possible.

- I/We request that our baby be handed immediately after delivery to his / her mother or father depending on the circumstances.   ☐ Yes   ☐ No

Fig. 1. Palliative care plan. *Adapted from* National Consensus Project for Quality Palliative Care, Editor Brandt, K. Clinical Practice Guidelines for Quality Palliative Care. Available at: https://www.nationalcoalitionhpc.org/wp-content/uploads/2020/07/NCHPC-NCPGuidelines_4thED_web_FINAL.pdf. Accessed June 22, 2021.

plans, intensive life-saving treatments may be initiated with the intention of gaining physiologic stability until full assessments can be completed.[3] At the end of life, infants in the NICU experience substantial symptoms, such as pain, dyspnea, agitation, and secretions.[29]

The NICU nurse must assess and manage those symptoms with standardized non-pharmacologic and pharmacologic guidelines established by the PPC team.[29] Non-pharmacologic measures include (1) non-nutritive sucking, (2) skin-to-skin interaction, (3) decreasing stimulation, and (4) repositioning. Medication classes used at the end of life include (1) opioids, (2) benzodiazepines, (3) antipyretics, (4) anticholinergics, (5) diuretics, (6) hypnotics, and (7) anticonvulsants[29] (**Table 2**). In the NICU setting, intravenous access typically is maintained as a way to provide these comfort medications.[29] NICU nurses require education and training in palliative care medication symptom management (Stenekes and colleagues[8]).

Because our baby may not survive for very long, please delay any procedures that can be put off until later. I/We want to have our baby in the room with us for all routine care. I/We request that as many routine and necessary procedures be performed with our baby in our arms.   ☐ Yes   ☐ No

- I/We request that a ceremony (blessing, baptism, etc) be performed in accordance with our religious beliefs by: _____   ☐ Yes   ☐ No

- I/We have arranged for a professional photographer to photograph our baby through_____   ☐ Yes   ☐ No

- I/We would like Woman's Hospital staff to photograph our baby.   ☐ Yes   ☐ No

- Special requests: _____

_____

_____

_____

Family Members

- I/We would like _____ to be present for delivery if possible.

- After delivery, I/we would like _____ to be able to come into our room and spend time with us and our baby.

- Special requests: _____

_____

_____

_____

Medical Management of the Infant

I/We have been informed of the natural history of our baby's diagnosis, and the poor prognosis associated with this condition.

If our baby is stillborn, I/we would like him / her to stay with us in our room for as long as possible.   ☐ Yes   ☐ No

If our baby is born alive:

☐ I/We wish to utilize all medical interventions available in order to prolong our baby's life.

OR

☐ I/We wish to utilize all medical interventions except _____ in order to prolong our baby's life.

OR

☐ I/We want no heroic measures, such as ventilation or resuscitation, to be initiated. I/We want our baby to receive medication to promote comfort but not to extend life. (Comfort care includes keeping baby warm, pain medication if necessary, feeding or other oral comfort measures.)

Fig. 1. (continued)

The NICU is a complex environment, and communication among the PPC health care team is challenging. The NICU nurse spends more time with the infant and the family than other PPC team health care providers and, therefore, is critical in the communication process for infants in palliative care.[21,30] This time factor fosters the relationship between the family and the NICU nurse and creates a level of trust.[21] This trust is evidenced by the family relying on the NICU nurse for support when care decisions need to be made or communication of the family needs to the care team.[21]

For the NICU nurse delivering palliative care to the infant and family, there are many key aspects requiring attention, including the following:

- The infant requires care with specific attention to detail much like any traditional NICU infant.

Feeding our baby:

•	I/We would like to attempt breast feeding	☐ Yes	☐ No
•	Bottle feeding formula	☐ Yes	☐ No
•	Bottle feeding breast milk	☐ Yes	☐ No
•	Feeding via dropper, NG or OG tubemay be used if our baby cannot suck or swallow.	☐ Yes	☐ No

Hospice Plans

If our baby survives longer than expected:

- I/We would like our baby in the room with us throughout our hospital stay with comfort measures provided for baby. ☐ Yes ☐ No

- I/We would like the baby to go to the NICU for comfort measures only. ☐ Yes ☐ No

- If baby survives longer than our expected hospital stay I/we would like hospice care to be arranged so that we can bring my baby home with us. ☐ Yes ☐ No

- If baby survives longer than our expected hospital stay I/we would like the infant transferred to an inpatient hospice. ☐ Yes ☐ No

Additional Testing

For the purpose of chromosome studies or other special testing to possibly determine a cause for our baby's condition please collect: (Check all that apply)

☐ Amniotic Fluid   ☐ Placental Tissue   ☐ Peripheral Blood   ☐ Cord Blood   ☐ Muscle Biopsy   ☐Nothing

End of life Care

Plans for our baby should his / her death occur prior to hospital discharge will include:

- Autopsy ☐ Yes ☐ No
- I /we would like the hospital to make arrangements for infant's remains. (We understand this is only possible if the infant is born without a heart rate, and is less than 20 weeks gestation). ☐ Yes ☐ No
- Funeral or private cremation arrangements have been made with _____ Funeral Home ☐ Yes ☐ No
- Other requests_____
- I/We have concerns about the cost of burial and would like information on financial assistance. ☐ Yes ☐ No
- Special Keepsakes Requested (Check all that apply)
  ☐ Bassinet card   ☐ Hats   ☐ ID bracelets   ☐ Photos   ☐ Handprints   ☐ Footprints
  ☐ Lock of Hair   ☐ Molds of hands and feet

- Other requests: _____

_____

_____

_____

Fig. 1. (continued)

- Vital signs are monitored, however, and extra care should be taken to minimize alarms or consider hands-on vital signs instead of using probes. Monitoring using arterial or umbilical lines may cease.
- Some diagnostic tests may be minimized, such as laboratory and radiographic tests.
- The use of some peripheral lines for medication and palliation may continue.
- Alternate medication delivery routes may be considered, but many are most effective when delivered intravenously. Intramuscular injections should be avoided.

<u>**Interdisciplinary Team Assembled**</u>

Member	Yes	No	Declined	Date
MFM	_____	_____	_____	_____
Neonatology	_____	_____	_____	_____
Social Worker	_____	_____	_____	_____
Hospice	_____	_____	_____	_____
NICU	_____	_____	_____	_____
Antepartum	_____	_____	_____	_____
Labor and Delivery	_____	_____	_____	_____

<u>**Signature of Parents:**</u>

We understand that this plan is meant to provide a guideline of our wishes for the delivery and care of our baby. Following this plan in its entirety may not be possible due to extenuating circumstances beyond our control.

_____   _____

Name   Date

_____   _____

Name   Date

This plan was completed after discussion with:

Name   Title   Date

_____

_____

_____

Fig. 1. (continued)

- Care, respect, and gentleness are used when removing any lines or life support apparatus.
- Parents may opt to be present when these lines and/or life support is removed. Human contact with family members should be encouraged while honoring family rituals and customs.[3]

Bereavement Care

The PPC team provides bereavement care by providing interventions that support the mother and family with the objective of decreasing feelings of grief, stress, and isolation.[5] During the PPC consult and care planning sessions, the parents are assessed for risk of grief, including (1) complicated, (2) disenfranchised, and/or (3) anticipatory.[21] In cases of multiples, when 1 infant does not survive, the intricate balance of dealing with the joy of birth and grief of death simultaneously requires attention because the grief process does not follow a traditional course.[31]

Complicated grief or persistent complex bereavement disorder goes beyond a normal grief period and the person assumes their life is irreparably damaged and that they cannot imagine that they can ever feel better.[32] Disenfranchised grief is the experience of losing or mourning the loss of a person, but the person was unable to properly grieve.[33] Anticipatory grief results in pain and sorrow and manifests when someone is seriously ill or dying.[34]

Table 2
Neonatal palliative care pharmacologic medications

Medication	Class	Symptom
Acetaminophen	COX-2 inhibitor	Fever, mild pain
Atropine	Anticholinergic	Secretions
Dexmedetomidine	Selective α_2-agonist	Agitation, pain
Fentanyl	Opioid	Pain, dyspnea
Gabapentin	Anticonvulsant	Agitation, neuroirritability
Glycopyrrolate	Anticholinergic	Secretions
Ketamine	Dissociative anesthetic	Agitation, pain
Lorazepam	Benzodiazepine	Agitation, dyspnea
Methadone	Opioid	Pain
Midazolam	Benzodiazepine	Agitation, dyspnea
Morphine	Opioid	Pain, dyspnea, agitation

Adapted from: Cortezzo DE, Meyer M. Neonatal end-of-life symptom management. Front. Pediatr. 2020; 8:574121. https://doi.org/10.3389/fped.2020.574121.

Based on the ongoing assessment of the family, a plan is developed to support the family and extended family. The NICU nurses must be part of the plan and bereavement care delivery. Because bereavement care is emotionally challenging, the NICU nursing staff should receive continual support for delivering palliative and bereavement care.[5] The following are offerings that should be performed in the NICU, including

- Anticipatory direction about the grieving process that includes the mother, father, and other family members
- Participation in bereavement rituals that meet the family's spiritual, religious, and cultural preferences
- Psychosocial support for entire family, including siblings
- Transparent and seamless communication between all of the care units involved in the perinatal bereavement care plan
- Peer-to-peer support and/or referral to community or Internet resources[5]
- Having access to an ethics committee should there be conflict regarding end-of-life decisions
- Should the baby get discharged home for palliative/hospice care, the family receives both practical and psychological support to prepare them for discharge.[5]

Moral Distress

NICU nurses that care for dying infants are subject to sadness and grief.[14] Moral distress is widespread in NICU setting, where decisions regarding end-of-life care and medical futility are prevalent.[35] The NICU nurse is confronted with dealing with enormous amounts of grief in dealing with the infants and families in PPC.[36] The loss of an infant can be referred to as traumatic grief.[36] The NICU nurse can be impacted negatively with compassion fatigue by caring for the infant and assisting families during these intense and often lengthy periods of grief.[36] Although the advances in medical technology have allowed the smallest and very ill infants to survive, the NICU nurse is left with moral and ethical considerations for the infant and family.[35]

Delivering ongoing care to infants and families requiring PPC has a cumulative stress effect on the NICU that may lead to moral distress and ultimately burnout.[37]

Moral distress often is inevitable, considering the frequency with which NICU nurses care for dying infants, manage the death process, and support families in the presence of staffing shortages, long worked hours, and work-life imbalance.[37,38]

A systematic review of health care provider perspectives regarding caring for infants receiving palliative care described how the NICU nurse rarely feels part of decision-making process but is focused primarily on providing support and education to families, which contributes to moral distress.[14]

As a result of experiencing the trauma experienced by parents, compassion fatigue and secondary traumatic stress disorder have been described when the health care team actually experiences the phenomenon of countertransference.[38] Delivering palliative care has been shown to create an environment of increased stress, burnout, and turnover.[38] This moral distress is exacerbated when a NICU nurse may care for this baby for months.[39]

IMPROVING PERINATAL PALLIATIVE CARE PROGRAMS IN THE NEONATAL INTENSIVE CARE UNIT

There have been many advancements to improve the delivery of PPC, including the development of protocols, pathways, education and training, and strategies to improve resilience[19] Dickson.[40] Being mindful of diverse cultures at this critical time assists the NICU nurse in delivering the most appropriate care in the form of rituals and memory making (Dickson[40]). Creating an environment in the NICU that supports the infant in PPC improves the delivery of care and supports the NICU nurse in the process.[19] NICU nurses described the facilitators of quality palliative care as (1) leadership, (2) clinical knowledge, and (3) morals, values, and beliefs.[15]

Palliative Care Guidelines

In multiple studies, NICU nurses describe the need for more formalized guidelines for the delivery of palliative care to infants.[14] In a survey investigating the confidence in palliative care delivery to infants, formal palliative care guidelines were associated with a higher level of confidence.[40,41] There are multiple resources that provide information and guidance to assist in the development of PPC guidelines, protocols, and potential resources.

In 2014, the Royal College of Paediatrics and Child Health published *Practical Guidance for the Management of Palliative Care on Neonatal Units* that provide solutions to the following 5 difficult questions for PPC providers

1. How should the infant be managed once a decision has been made to withdraw or withhold life-sustaining treatments?
2. How should conflicts about end-of-life decisions on the neonatal unit be resolved in practice?
3. What support should be offered to parents and families once palliative care is instituted for an infant, and what bereavement support should be provided?
4. What is good practice in relation to seeking consent for postmortem examination and organ donation in infants?
5. What support is needed by staff to help them manage an infant receiving palliative care?

In 2017, Together for Short Lives produced *A Perinatal Pathway for Babies with Palliative Care Needs*, describing a framework of 3 stages consisting of 6 standards[41–43]:

- Stage 1: recognition of a life-limiting condition
  - Standard 1: sharing significant news

○ Standard 2: planning for choice in the location of care
- Stage 2: ongoing care
  ○ Standard 3: a multiagency assessment of family needs
  ○ Standard 4: coordinated multiagency care plans
- Stage 3: end-of-life bereavement care
  ○ Standard 5: an end-of-life care plan
  ○ Standard 6: continuing bereavement support and care

This document is one that provides a substantive framework for developing a protocol for PPC, including relevant research, case studies, and resources (Together for Short Lives).

For organizations developing a palliative care program, there are multiple resources that provide evidence-based guidance. Regardless of the type of care protocols that are developed, quality metrics, including process and outcome data, should be developed and reviewed on a regular basis.[22] Debriefing, document audits, and education are integral processes of a robust PPC program.[22] With availability of multiple resources, PPC programs often are not as mature as are adult and child palliative care programs.[22] Palliative care guidelines and protocols reduce ethical dilemmas and provide a framework for consistently providing palliative care to infants requiring end-of-life care.[19]

Memory Making and Legacy

Memory-making practices are a significant intervention for families and include both physical artifacts and caregiving activities.[44–46] Whether the loss is anticipated or unanticipated, the NICU nurse often is interacting on a continual basis with the family and facilitates efforts to have the family involved in decision making and memory making. Memory-making activities, such as handprints and footprints, photography, and keepsake boxes, often are performed and/or assisted by the NICU nurse[5,26] (**Fig. 2**). Parents report that they value guidance and support from the NICU nurse in taking part in memory-making projects and caregiving activities.[44] Families also may seek solace in having clothes or some care items used by their infant as mementos.[44]

Families may seek to create a lasting legacy for their infant. These activities may include organ/tissue donation, breast milk donation, and contributions to research.[26] Special considerations must be instituted in cases of multiple births when 1 infant does not survive.[31] Families want their twins or multiples to have time together.[31] All efforts for memory making that include their infants together are favorable.[31] NICU nurses should have a comprehensive list of possible memory-making activities available.[46]

Perinatal Palliative Education

To improve the care to dying infants, NICU nurses describe the need for more palliative care education.[14,47] For the physicians who ultimately lead these PPC care teams, there is a lack of training in palliative care in neonatal or perinatal medicine fellowship programs.[16]

Since 2000, the End-of-Life Nursing Education Consortium (ELNEC) has been an international education project that has provided opportunities to improve palliative care.[48] As of April 2021, there were more than 40,000 nurses and health care professionals in more than 50 states and 100 international locations who have completed the train-the-trainer course (ELNEC Fact Sheet).[48] Many states, however, have only a few health care professionals prepared at this level, and there are fewer than 300 trained at

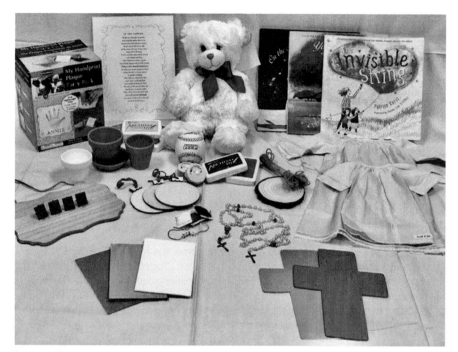

Fig. 2. Palliative care memory making.

this level in the United States.[49] Even fewer are those certified in pediatrics.[49] The pediatric certification contains perinatal and neonatal palliative care content.[48]

Palliative care education for the NICU nurse from ELNEC includes recognizing those infant diagnoses that could benefit from supportive palliative care.[21] This is of particular relevance when there is an unexpected preterm delivery of a previable infant.[21] When an infant has a potentially life-limiting illness, it may be appropriate for NICU nurses to advocate for infants who are extremely ill to receive palliative care while waiting for genetic testing to be completed.[21] Finally, the NICU nurse should be able to recognize and advocate for palliative care when neonatal intensive care interventions appear futile.[21]

Fostering Resilience

New evidence has emerged regarding a mindfulness-based, psychosocial framework to assist providers in dealing with families experiencing traumatic grief.[36] Health care organizations providing PPC need to provide programs and develop leadership to improve resilience.[37] Cacciatore[36] described the ATTEND (attunement, trust, touch, egalitarianism, nuance, and death education) framework that promotes mindful caregiver feelings and behaviors that assist both provider and family.[50] Some of the techniques employed include meditation and teaching mind-body awareness (Cacciatore[36]). Meditation may provide an alternative for caring for bereaved parents; it may assist providers of the PPC team relief from moral distress (Cacciatore[36]).

In the NICU, when delivering PPC, nurses practicing self-care may build resilience in the presence of perceived immense suffering and loss.[38] Development of self-care plans are more vigorous and serve as a model for others about the importance of self-compassion and care.[38] A comprehensive intentional self-care plan improves empathy.[38] These plans need to be individualized to the preferences of the NICU nurse, which can include exercise and journaling.[38] Journaling or self-reflective writing allows the NICU nurse to partake in a practice of critically examining the dilemmas of individual PPC infants, which can assist in improving resiliency.[35] Finally, due to the frequent ethical dilemmas encountered by the NICU nurse, ethics training has been effective in improving resilience.[35]

Environmental Considerations

The NICU nurse can have a positive impact the physical environment in the selection and preparation of an area appropriate for neonatal palliative care.[19] Providing a home-like atmosphere with soft lighting and sufficient space for the extended family is desired.[19] Ideally, there is access to kitchen facilities, and the provision of recliners or beds for parents is optimal.[19] Access to a nearby conference room, chapel, and/or library comprises other environmental considerations for PPC programs.[19] In certain situations, the parents may request for their infant to not be in the NICU and be in an adjoining patient care unit, requiring the NICU nurse to deliver care elsewhere in the hospital (Mancini and colleagues[40]).

Should the parents choose to take their infant home, the NICU nurse is instrumental in delivering parental education during this transition (Together for Short Lives). The parents should be able to access to the interdisciplinary plan of care and be able to take this home (Together for Short Lives). The NICU nurse is instrumental in facilitating the transition to home care. Providing support by phone to the family is in the scope of care that the NICU nurse delivers.

Future Research

Because PPC still is evolving as a specialty, more research is required to develop programs that meet the comprehensive needs of the infant, families, and care providers. Research needs to include studies to objectively quantify the knowledge of the participants in PPC educational programs.[13] Approaches by providers, such as mindfulness practices, that may assist families undergoing traumatic grief should be studied further.[36] Additional qualitative studies should be performed to further describe perceptions of care by neonatal advanced practice registered nurses.[14] Outcome-related data are needed related to nurses' level of comfort with providing neonatal palliative care after obtaining specific ELNEC training using the evidence-based curriculum.[21]

DISCUSSION

PPC is a relatively new palliative care phenomenon in the NICU. Creating a comprehensive PPC program requires (1) interdisciplinary team effort, (2) well-developed protocols, (3) detailed individualized care plans, (4) environmental considerations, (5) extensive education and training, and (6) resilience-building activities. The NICU nurse often spends more time with the infant and families than do other providers and, therefore, is pivotal to improving the PPC experience. Therefore, the NICU nurse is in a unique position to improve the outcomes of PPC programs.

DISCLOSURE

The author has nothing to disclose.

REFERENCES

1. Limbo R, Lathrop A, Heustis J. Caregiving as a theoretical framework in perinatal palliative care. In: Black BP, Wright PM, Limbo R, editors. Perinatal and pediatric

bereavement: in nursing and other health professions. New York: Springer; 2016. p. 33–55.

2. Ely DM, Driscoll AK. Infant mortality in the United States, 2018: data from the period linked birth/infant death file. In: National vital statistics reports 2020; 69 (7). Available at: https://www.cdc.gov/nchs/data/nvsr/nvsr69/NVSR-69-7-508. pdf. Accessed April 12, 2021.

3. Kuelbelbeck A, Carter B. Exploring the concept of palliative care for babies and their families. In: Mancini A, Price J, Kerr-Elliot T, editors. Neonatal palliative care for nurses. Cham (Switzerland): Springer; 2020. p. 9–20.

4. Abramson P, Mancini A. The importance of effective communication on a neonatal unit. In: Mancini A, Price J, Kerr-Elliot T, editors. Neonatal palliative care for nurses. Cham (Switzerland): Springer; 2020. p. 39–57.

5. Kenner C, Press J, Ryan D. Recommendations for palliative and bereavement care in the NICU: a family-centered integrative approach. J Perinatalogy 2015; 35:519–23.

6. Carter BS. Pediatric palliative care in infants and neonates. Children 2018;5(21). Available at: https://www.ncbi.nlm.nih.gov/pmc/articles/PMC5835990/pdf/children-05-00021.pdf. Accessed April 12, 2021.

7. Kiman R, Doumic L. Perinatal palliative care: a developing specialty. Int J Palliat Nurs 2014;20(3):143–8.

8. Stenekes S, Penner JL, Harlos M, et al. Development and implementation of a survey to assess health-care provider's competency, attitudes, and knowledge about perinatal palliative care. J Palliat Care 2019;34(3):151–9.

9. Leuthner SR. Fetal palliative care. Clin Perinatol 2004;31(3):649–55.

10. Cole A, Craig F, Daly C, et al. Palliative care (supportive and end of life care) a framework for clinical practice in perinatal medicine. In: British association of perinatal medicine (BAPM). 2010. Available at: https://hubble-live-assets.s3.amazonaws.com/bapm/attachment/file/38/Palliative_care_final_version__Aug10.pdf. Accessed June 16, 2021.

11. Flaig F, Lotz JD, Knochel K, et al. Perinatal palliative care: a qualitative study evaluating the perspectives of pregnancy counselors. Palliat Med 2019;33(6):704–11.

12. Hasegawa SL, Fry JT. Moving toward a shared process: the impact of parent experiences on perinatal palliative care. Semin Perinatology 2017;41:95–100.

13. Ratislavova K, Buzgova R, Vejvodova J. Perinatal palliative care education: an integrative review. Nurse Education Today 2019;82:58–66.

14. Beltran SJ, Hamel MN. Caring for dying infants: a systematic review of healthcare providers' perspectives of neonatal palliative care. Am J Hosp Palliat Med 2020;1–15.

15. Kilcullen M, Ireland S. Palliative care in the neonatal unit: neonatal nursing staff perceptions of facilitators and barriers in a regional tertiary nursery. BMC Palliat Care 2017;16(32):1–12.

16. Forman KR, Thomson-Branch A. Educational perspectives: palliative care education in neonatal-perinatal medicine fellowship. NeoReviews 2020;21:72–9.

17. Brandt MS. Clinical practice guidelines for quality palliative care. National Consensus Project for Quality Palliative Care; 2018. Available at: https://www.nationalcoalitionhpc.org/wp-content/uploads/2020/07/NCHPC-NCPGuidelines_4thED_web_FINAL.pdf. Accessed June 22, 2021.

18. Palliative care. In: Newsroom Fact sheets. World Health Organization. 2020. Available at: https://www.who.int/news-room/fact-sheets/detail/palliative-care. Accessed July 11, 2021.

19. Catlin A, Carter B. Creation of a neonatal end-of-life palliative care protocol. J Perinatology 2002. Available at: http://www.icpcn.org/wp-content/uploads/2018/06/Creation-of-a-neonatal-EOLPC-protocol.pdf. Accessed June 17, 2021.
20. Limbo R, Wool C. Perinatal palliative care. Available at: https://www.jognn.org/action/showPdf?pii=S0884-2175%2816%2930279-9. Accessed June 22, 2021.
21. Ferrell B, Thaxton CA, Murphy H. Preparing nurses for palliative care in the NICU. Adv Neonatal Care 2020;20(2):142–50.
22. Lago P, Cavicchiolo ME, Rusalen F, et al. Summary of the key concepts on how to develop a perinatal palliative care program. Front Pediatr 2020;8:596744.
23. Palliative (end of life) neonatal care. In: Victorian agency for health information. Available at: https://www.bettersafercare.vic.gov.au/clinical-guidance/neonatal/palliative-end-of-life-neonatal-care#goto-more-information. Accessed June 28, 2021.
24. Niehaus JZ, Palmer MM, Slaven J, et al. Neonatal palliative care: perception differences between providers. J Perinatology 2020;40:1802–8.
25. Sidgwick P, Harrop E, Kelly B, et al. Fifteen-minute consultation: perinatal palliative care. Arch Dis Child Educ Prac Ed 2017;102(3):114–6.
26. Cortezzo DE, Ellis K, Schegel A. Perinatal palliative care birth planning as advance care planning. Front Pediatr 2020;8:556.
27. Quinn M, Weiss AB, Crist JD. Early for everyone: reconceptualizing palliative care in the neonatal intensive care unit. Adv Neonatal Care 2020;20(2):109–17.
28. Palliative and end-of-life care for newborns and infants. Position statement # 3063. Neonatal Association of Neonatal Nurses. 2015. Available at: http://nann.org/uploads/About/PositionPDFS/1.4.5_Palliative%20and%20End%20of%20Life%20Care%20for%20Newborns%20and%20Infants.pdf. Accessed April 12, 2021.
29. Cortezzo DE, Meyer M. Neonatal end-of-life symptom management. Front Pediatr 2020;8:574121.
30. Falck AJ, Moorthy S, Hussey-Gardner B. Perceptions of palliative care in the NICU. Available at: file:///C:/Users/qa-cmg/Downloads/Perceptions_of_Palliative_Care_in_the_NICU.7.pdf. Accessed April 12, 2021.
31. Campbell C. Care of twins, multiple births and support for the family: a detailed background. In: Mancini A, Price J, Kerr-Elliot T, editors. Neonatal palliative care for nurses. Cham (Switzerland): Springer; 2020. p. 155–75.
32. Complicated grief. The center for complicated grief. Available at: https://complicatedgrief.columbia.edu/for-the-public/complicated-grief-public/overview/. Accessed July 2, 2021.
33. Disenfranchised grief: mourning events that never were. Psychology Today. Available at: https://www.psychologytoday.com/us/blog/lifetime-connections/202103/disenfranchised-grief-mourning-events-never-were. Accessed July 2, 2021.
34. Anticipatory grief. Kansas City hospice and palliative care. Available at: https://www.kchospice.org/family/caregiver-tips/anticipatory-grief/. Accessed July 2, 2021.
35. Mills M, Cortezzo DE. Moral distress in the neonatal intensive care unit: what is it, why it happens, and how can we address it. Front Pediatr 2020;8:581.
36. Cacciatore J. When the unthinkable happens: a mindfulness approach to perinatal and pediatric death. In: Black BP, Wright PM, Limbo R, editors. Perinatal and pediatric bereavement: in nursing and other health professions. New York: Springer; 2016. p. 97–110.

37. Black R, Honeyman A. Support for staff: building resilience in nurses. In: Mancini A, Price J, Kerr-Elliot T, editors. Neonatal palliative care for nurses. New York: Springer; 2020. p. 21–38.

38. Grauerholz KR, Fredenburg M, Jones PT, et al. Fostering vicarious resilience for perinatal palliative care professionals. Front Pediatr 2020;8:572933.

39. Limbo R, Kobler K. Moments matter: exploring the evidence of caring for grieving families and self. In: Black BP, Wright PM, Limbo R, editors. Perinatal and pediatric bereavement: in nursing and other health professions. New York: Springer; 2016.

40. Dickson G. A perinatal pathway for babies with palliative care needs. In: Chambers L, Dickson G, Detzler S, editors. Together for short lives. 2017. Available at: https://www.togetherforshortlives.org.uk/wp-content/uploads/2018/01/ProRes-Perinatal-Pathway-for-Babies-With-Palliative-Care-Needs.pdf. Accessed July 11, 2021.

41. Wool C. Clinician confidence and comfort in providing perinatal palliative care. J Obstet Gynecol Neonatal Nurs 2013;42(1):48–58.

42. Mancini A, Uthaya S, Beardsley C, et al. Practical guidance for the management of palliative care on neonatal units. 1st edition. Royal College of Peadiatrics and Child Health; 2014. Available at: file:///C:/Users/qa-cmg/Downloads/ExRes_NICU-Palliative-Care-Feb-2014.pdf. Accessed on April 16, 2021.

43. American College of Obstetricians and Gynecologists. Perinatal palliative care. Committee opinion No. 786. Washington (DC): American College of Obstetricians and Gynecologists; 2019. Available at: https://www.acog.org/-/media/project/acog/acogorg/clinical/files/committee-opinion/articles/2019/09/perinatal-palliative-care.pdf. Accessed May 7, 2021.

44. Thornton R, Nicholson P, Harms L. Scoping review of memory making in bereavement care for parents after the death of a newborn. J Obstet Gynecol Neonatal Nurs 2019;48:351–60.

45. Marc-Aurele KL. Decisions parents make when faced with potentially life-limiting fetal diagnoses and the importance of perinatal palliative care. Front Pediatr 2020;8:574556.

46. Bereavement interventions that NICU staff can offer parents. Support 4 NICU Parents. Available at: https://support4nicuparents.org/wp-content/uploads/2016/04/Bereavement-Interventions-that-NICU-Staff-Can-Offer-Parents.pdf. Accessed July 20, 2021.

47. Catlin A, Brandon D, Wool C, et al. Palliative and end-of-life care for newborns and infants. Advances in neonatal care. 2015. Available at: file:///C:/Users/qa-cmg/Downloads/Palliative_and_End_of_Life_Care_for_Newborns_and.5.pdf. Accessed April 12, 2021.

48. Fact sheet. End-of-life nursing education consortium (ELNEC). April 2021. Available at: https://www.aacnnursing.org/Portals/42/ELNEC/PDF/ELNEC-Fact-Sheet.pdf. Accessed July 1, 2021.

49. Find a trainer. End-of-life nursing education consortium (ELNEC). Available at: https://www.aacnnursing.org/ELNEC/Tools-for-Trainers/Find-a-Trainer. Accessed July 1, 2021.

50. Cacciatore J. Stillbirth: clinical recommendations for care in the era of evidence-based medicine. Clin Obstet Gynecol 2010;53(3):691–9.

Palliative Care and Dementia

What All Advanced Practice Nurses Should Know

Phyllis Whitehead, PhD, APRN/CNS, ACHPN, PMGT-BC, FNAP, FAAN[a,b,*]

KEYWORDS

- Dementia • Palliative care • Hospice • Advanced practice nurses
- Advance care planning

KEY POINTS

- Patients and families do not understand that dementia is a life-limiting/terminal condition that should be discussed early so patients' preferences align with their treatments and interventions as the disease progresses.
- Palliative care APRNs should engage early with communication about goal setting in the face of dementia management and can help to align patient and provider expectations with the reality of living with dementia.
- Team-based care, such as palliative care and hospice, is essential to address patients' and families' needs.

INTRODUCTION

The incidence of dementia is growing especially with the baby boomers aging. It occurs in approximately 1% of all people 65 years of age and 50% of people aged 90 years. Worldwide, 24 million individuals are living with dementia, and this number is predicted to double over the next 20 years.[1,2] Dementia, specifically Alzheimer disease, is the fifth leading cause of death.[3,4] Dementia is a progressive, incurable condition that causes limitations in life and should be recognized as a life-limiting condition.[4]

Dementia is a common diagnosis seen in palliative medicine in acute and primary care settings.[5] Frequently, families do not understand that dementia is a life-limiting/terminal condition that should be discussed early so patients' preferences align their treatments and interventions as the disease progresses. Advanced practice registered nurses (APRNs), such as clinical nurse specialists and nurse practitioners,

[a] Carilion Roanoke Memorial Hospital Palliative Care Service, 1906 Belleview Avenue Southeast, Roanoke, VA 24014, USA; [b] Virginia Tech Carilion School of Medicine, 2 Riverside Circle, Roanoke, VA 24014, USA
* Carilion Roanoke Memorial Hospital Palliative Care Service, 1906 Belleview Avenue Southeast, Roanoke, VA 24014.
E-mail address: pbwhitehead@carilionclinic.org

Crit Care Nurs Clin N Am 34 (2022) 121–127
https://doi.org/10.1016/j.cnc.2021.11.005
0899-5885/22/© 2021 Elsevier Inc. All rights reserved.
ccnursing.theclinics.com

are uniquely positioned to initiate conversations to help families understand the disease trajectory for patients with dementia.[6]

HISTORY/DEFINITIONS/BACKGROUND

Dementia can have many causes, such as Alzheimer disease, vascular dementia, advanced Parkinson or Huntington disease, Lewy body disease, and excessive and chronic alcohol use.[3] Impairments in mental and physical functioning, such as memory loss, language impairment, personality changes, dysphagia, and inability to perform activities of daily living, characterize the condition.[7] There are seven stages of dementia (**Table 1**). The APRN should be familiar with these stages to guide patients, health care professionals (HCPs), and families to understand the role of palliative and hospice care for patients and their loved ones.

The terms palliative care and hospice care are often used interchangeably for one another, yet there is a significant difference between the two patient services. The National Hospice and Palliative Care Organization, Hospice and Palliative Nurses Association, and the American Academy of Hospice and Palliative Medicine clearly state that palliative care is not hospice care.[10,11] Palliative care does not replace the patient's primary treatment being received. It focuses on pain, symptoms, and stress of serious illness most often as an adjunct to curative care modalities. The National Cancer Institute's definition of palliative care is defined as care given to improve the quality of life of patients who have a serious or chronic disease, such as cancer. Palliative care is an approach to care that addresses the person as a whole, not just a disease. The goal is to prevent or treat, as early as possible, the symptoms and side effects of the disease and treatments, in addition to any related psychological, social, and spiritual challenges.[12]

Hospice care is defined is services focusing on pain, symptoms, and distress at the end-stage of a serious illness. The terminal phase is defined by Medicare as an individual with a life expectancy of 6 months or less of the illness, disease, or condition. The critical differences between palliative care and hospice care are the time limitation and not pursuing aggressive interventions in hospice. Whereas hospice care is provided when life expectancy is 6 months or less, palliative care has no time limitation

Table 1 Stages of dementia	
Stage	**Impairment Level**
1	No impairment
2	Very mild decline – unnoticeable memory lapses
3	Mild decline – noticeable memory and concentration problems Losing items
4	Moderate decline – forgetfulness of events Difficulty performing tasks
5	Moderate to severe decline – gaps in memory, thinking Needs help with activities of daily living
6	Severe decline – loss of awareness of recent experiences Remembers own name but has difficulty with others
7	Very severe decline – total care Impaired swallowing Hospice eligible

Adapted from Refs.[8,9]

and may be elected to manage secondary symptoms resulting from treatments for illness of which recovery is a possible, but not guaranteed.[13]

Palliative medicine provides a team-based approach to patient care integrating comprehensive assessment of patient needs and addressing needs across a variety of domains: (1) management of pain, symptoms, and side effects of treatments; (2) caregiver support; (3) social support; and (4) spiritual support. Addressing these domains may lead to improvement in pain and symptom management and relief of psychological, emotional, and spiritual suffering.[10,14] When caring for patients diagnosed with dementia, family and caregiver support is paramount and includes referrals to local community resources as indicated to allow better, more individualized care for patients in their preferred environment, whether that be home, long-term care, or group home settings.[15]

Palliative care APRNs should engage early with communication about goal setting in the face of dementia management and can help to align patient and provider expectations with the reality of living with dementia. Team-based care is usually provided by physicians/providers, nurses, social workers, and chaplains, but also possibly including dieticians, counselors/psychologists, pharmacists, therapists (physical, occupational, or speech), and volunteers.[16]

DISCUSSION

A common challenge for HCPs is the difficulty of identifying dementia as a life-limiting illness and importance of obtaining appropriate palliative care consultation for the patient. Evidence shows patients with end-stage dementia are less likely to be referred to palliative care than other nononcologic end-stage disease patients (9% vs 25%), and patients with dementia are likely to be prescribed fewer palliative medications (28% vs 51%).[3] Caregivers' burden is worsened when periods of stability are interrupted by acute exacerbations, in contrast to the more predictable decline in patients with advanced cancer. Advance care planning and goal setting should be initiated early in the disease progression, while the patient can provide guidance to their caregivers and families. Because of the progression of dementia, it is challenging for family and HCPs to know when to initiate palliation as a goal. The use of functionality and cognition scales, such as the Minimum Data Set 2 or the Functional Assessment Staging instruments, is helpful in quantifying the stage and identifying appropriate palliative and/or hospice patients.[2,8,17]

Pain (39%) and dyspnea (46%) are common symptoms at end-of-life for many patients with dementia.[6] Patients with dementia receive less analgesia than patients who are cognitively intact. They often cannot express themselves verbally and hence receive suboptimal palliation. These symptoms should be aggressively treated as recommended with an opioid, such as morphine. Behavioral pain assessment tools, such as the Pain Assessment in Advanced Dementia Scale, should be integrated as part of a comprehensive assessment with patients with advanced dementia. The American Society of Pain Management Nursing's "Position Statement on Pain Assessment in Patients Unable to Self-Report" recommends using patient self-report of pain if possible, review of known pain etiologies from the medical history, observation of pain-related behaviors, and family or proxy reports to assess for pain in the patient with dementia.[18] Agitation may affect up to half of patients with end-stage dementia, necessitating a calm environment and the treatment of reversible causes, such as pain, dyspnea, and constipation.[19,20]

The APRN should assess for cognitive changes, including delirium. Such tools as the Mini-Mental State Examination, the Short Portable Mental Status Questionnaire, the

Delirium Observation Screening Scale, and the Confusion Assessment Method are used to screen for cognitive changes and delirium to enhance symptom management.[18,21]

Infections, such as pneumonia from aspiration, urinary tract infections, or pressure ulcers from lack of mobility, are a natural part of the disease progression. The APRN should anticipate these infections and proactively discuss with caregivers the role of antibiotics in the context of a life-prolonging intervention, especially in the late stages of the disease. Antibiotics are not benign and can cause complications, such as *Clostridium difficile* infection, so an early dialogue is warranted about the use of oral and/or intravenous antibiotics as contingent on the patient's goals of care with an understanding that they will becoming life prolonging and nonbeneficial.[2,21]

Because of the prevalence of dysphagia (93%), malnutrition and dehydration are common. Conversations on the use of artificial hydration and nutrition should start early and continue as the disease progresses.[15] There are many resources, such as the video from the University of North Carolina School of Medicine Palliative Care Resources on feeding options (http://www.med.unc.edu/pcare/resources/feedingoptions), to provide patients and their caregivers with accurate information on the benefits and risks of artificial nutrition versus careful hand feeding so patients and their caregivers can make informed decisions. A speech-language pathologist referral may be considered to determine the safest oral intake/diet recommendations for the patient.[22,23]

Frequently, caregivers struggle with the determining the right course of care and ask how we can allow the patient to "starve to death." A candid discussion on the natural dying process for a patient with dementia is imperative. Using careful selection of words, such as "fasting," and explaining that this process is not uncomfortable, is helpful for caregivers. Comparing the fasting state with a time when the loved one has been ill and did not have a desire to eat may also be helpful. It is important to emphasize the patient will be offered comfort foods and/or sips of beverages, despite the risk of aspiration, along with frequent oral care. Providing the information and allowing caregivers time to process while providing empathy are essential APRN skills.[2]

ADVANCE CARE PLANNING

The Institute of Medicine report "Dying in America: Improving Quality and Honoring Individual Preferences Near the End of Life" recommends that HCPs encourage Advance Care Planning (ACP) conversations throughout the disease trajectory as long as the patient has capacity to do so. They emphasize the importance of documentation, such advance directives.[24] ACP is a process that encourages persons of all ages dealing with serious illness to understand, identify, and share their values, goals, and preferences regarding future medical care.[17,25,26]

Because seriously ill patients with dementia lose their decision-making capacity, the HCP may have to rely on loved ones to advocate for the patient's wishes. State laws vary in the extent to which they authorize proxy decision making; they also differ as to which family members have priority in the decision making. Thus, the APRN should be familiar with the state's surrogate decision-making laws and regulations. The APRN should initiate family meetings early within the disease trajectory, so the patient can appoint a surrogate decision maker for health care decisions and share care preferences with the surrogate. ACP conversations should occur to ensure surrogates understand the patient's priorities of care to align future treatment plans. APRNs should start early with ACP conversations and they should be ongoing as the patient's condition progresses.[1]

Patient and family meetings are crucial interventions in establishing goals of care for patients. During the patient and family meeting, the APRN needs to provide an accurate summary of the medical care to date; the potential medical treatment options that may be considered in the future, especially the use of artificial hydration and nutrition at end of life; and the potential outcomes, including prognosis.

In the acute care setting, the APRN should summarize what the medical teams are recommending as the best care options, while focusing on the patient's preferences and values. For example, "In light of what we have talked about so far, what do you think your loved one would want to do?" The goals of the meeting are to minimize the surrogate decision maker's burden of responsibility and to remain focused on the patient's wishes, not the decision maker's wishes.

Once ACP decisions have been made it is crucial to document treatment preferences in one of the many advance directive documents, such as Five Wishes, POLST/POST/MOST, and DDNAR to mention a few. These documents need to be shared with all HCPs and facilities.[3]

With most deaths occurring in acute care settings, where the focus of care is on active, curative treatment and not on managing symptoms or establishing realistic goals of care, APRNs must be able to advocate for seriously ill patients and their loved ones. Patients need HCPs who are skilled in the science of palliation and skilled ACP and the art of holistic healing. With the ever-changing health care environment, APRNs are essential in providing specialized interventions to meet the diverse needs of acute care patients.[27,28]

SUMMARY

Caring for patients with dementia continues to be challenging. It is imperative that APRNs initiate goals of care conversations early with the patient to better understand treatment preferences. Additionally, early integration of palliative medicine can better manage symptoms and lessen the strain on loved ones. Palliative medicine APRNs should be a standardized part of treatment for patients who are diagnosed with dementia. Finally, early enrollment into hospice should be discussed with loved ones as an intervention in promoting quality of life for these patients and their loved ones. APRNs can and should provide more comprehensive care and support for their patients diagnosed with dementia. This includes early and ongoing advance care planning. This is accomplished in partnership with palliative medicine and hospice.

CLINICS CARE POINTS

- Dementia, specifically Alzheimer disease, is the fifth leading cause of death. Patients and families do not understand that dementia is a life-limiting/terminal condition that should be discussed early so patients' preferences align with their treatments and interventions as the disease progresses.

- Palliative care APRNs should engage early with communication about goal setting in the face of dementia management and can help to align patient and provider expectations with the reality of living with dementia. Team-based care is needed. This is usually provided by physicians, advanced practice nurses, nurses, social workers, and chaplains, but should also include dieticians, counselors/psychologists, pharmacists, therapists (physical, occupational, or speech), and volunteers.

DISCLOSURE

The author has no actual or potential conflicts.

REFERENCES

1. Sommerbakk R, Haugen DF, Tjora A, et al. Barriers to and facilitators for implementing quality improvements in palliative care: results from a qualitative interview study in Norway. BMC Palliat Care 2016;15(1):61. https://doi.org/10.1186/s12904-016-0132-5.
2. Ernecoff NC, Wessell KL, Hanson LC, et al. Does receipt of recommended elements of palliative care precede in-hospital death or hospice referral? J Pain Symptom Manage 2020;59(4):778–86. https://doi.org/10.1016/j.jpainsymman.2019.11.011.
3. Burns RB, Waikar SS, Wachterman MW, et al. Trends in hospital-based specialty palliative care in the United States from 2013 to 2017. J Pain Symptom Manage 2018;10(1):774–80. https://doi.org/10.1111/jocn.13925.
4. Burns RB, Waikar SS, Wachterman MW, et al. Management options for an older adult with advanced chronic kidney disease and dementia: grand rounds discussion from Beth Israel Deaconess Medical Center. Ann Intern Med 2020;173(3): 217–25. https://doi.org/10.7326/M20-2640.
5. Mo L, Geng Y, Chang YK, et al. Referral criteria to specialist palliative care for patients with dementia: a systematic review. J Am Geriatr Soc 2021. https://doi.org/10.1111/jgs.17070.
6. Kramarow EA, Tejada-Vera B. Dementia mortality in the United States, 2000-2017. Natl Vital Stat Rep 2019;68(2):1–29.
7. Joling KJ, Janssen O, Francke AL, et al. Time from diagnosis to institutionalization and death in people with dementia. Alzheimers Dement 2020;16(4):662–71.
8. Reisberg B. Functional assessment staging (FAST). Psychopharmacol Bull 1988; 24(4):653–9.
9. Hum A, Tay RY, Wong YKY, et al. Advanced dementia: an integrated homecare programme. BMJ Support Palliat Care 2019;0:1–10.
10. Whitehead PB, Dahlin C, editors. Compendium of nursing care for common serious illnesses. 3rd edition. Pittsburg: Hospice and Palliative Nurses Association; 2019.
11. Shah RJ, Korenstein D, Flynn JR, et al. Resource utilization in hospitalized patients with cancer from hospice decision to discharge and provider-type differences. Am J Hosp Palliat Med 2020;37(7):503–6. https://doi.org/10.1177/1049909119889289.
12. Shippee ND, Shippee TP, Mobley PD, et al. Effect of a whole-person model of care on patient experience in patients with complex chronic illness in late life. Am J Hosp Palliat Med 2018;35(1):104–9. https://doi.org/10.1177/1049909117690710.
13. Kang KA, Han SJ, Lim YS, et al. Meaning-centered interventions for patients with advanced or terminal cancer: a meta-analysis. Cancer Nurs 2019;42(4):332–40. https://doi.org/10.1097/NCC.0000000000000628.
14. Teo I, Krishnan A, Lee GL. Psychosocial interventions for advanced cancer patients: a systematic review. Psychooncology 2019;28(7):1394–407. https://doi.org/10.1002/pon.5103.
15. Ernecoff NC, Zimmerman S, Mitchell SL, et al. Concordance between goals of care and treatment decisions for person with dementia. J Palliat Med 2018; 21(10):1442–7.

16. Program C, Yosick L, Crook RE, et al. Effects of a population health community-based palliative care program on cost and utilization 2019;29(9):1075–81. https://doi.org/10.1089/jpm.2018.0489.

17. Scott J, Owen-Smith A, Tonkin-Crine S, et al. Decision-making for people with dementia and advanced kidney disease: a secondary qualitative analysis of interviews from the Conservative Kidney Management Assessment of Practice Patterns Study. BMJ Open 2018;8(11):e022385. https://doi.org/10.1136/bmjopen-2018-022385.

18. Herr K, Coyne PJ, Ely E, et al. Pain assessment in the patient unable to self-report: clinical practice recommendations in support of the ASPMN 2019 position statement. Pain Manag Nurs 2019;20(5):404–17. https://doi.org/10.1016/j.pmn.2019.07.005.

19. Herr K, Coyne PJ, Ely E, et al. ASPMN 2019 position statement: pain assessment in the patient unable to self-report. Pain Manag Nurs 2019;20:402–3. https://doi.org/10.1016/j.pmn.2019.07.007.

20. Bellile A, Whitehead PB. Pain management. In: Farinde A, Hebdon M, editors. Pharmacological considerations in gerontology: a patient-centered guide for advanced practice registered nurses and related health professions. New York: Springer Publishing Company; 2020. p. 211–26.

21. Gleason LJ, Benton EA, Alvarez-Nebreda ML, et al. FRAIL Questionnaire screening tool and short-term outcomes in geriatric fracture patients. J Am Med Dir Assoc 2017;18(12):1082–6. https://doi.org/10.1016/j.jamda.2017.07.005.

22. Eisenmann Y, Golla H, Schmidt H, et al. Palliative care in advanced dementia. Front Psychiatry 2020;11:699.

23. Hill E, Savundranayagam MY, Zecevic A, et al. Staff perspectives of barriers to access and delivery of palliative care for persons with dementia in long-term care. Am J Alzheimers Dis Other Demen 2018;33(5):284–91.

24. IOM (Institute of Medicine), Dying in America: Improving quality and honoring individual preferences near the end of life. Washington, DC; The National Academies Press. 2015, doi:10.17226/18748.

25. Ouchi K, George N, Revette AC, et al. Empower seriously ill older adults to formulate their goals for medical care in the emergency department. J Palliat Med 2018;22(3):267–73. https://doi.org/10.1089/jpm.2018.0360.

26. Forzley B, Er L, Chiu HHL, et al. External validation and clinical utility of a prediction model for 6-month mortality in patients undergoing hemodialysis for end-stage kidney disease. Palliat Med 2018;32(2):395–403. https://doi.org/10.1177/0269216317720832.

27. Bolt S, van der Steen J, Schols J, et al. What do relatives value most in end-of-life care for people with dementia? Int J Palliat Nurs 2019;25(9):432–42.

28. Hum A, Tay RY, Wong YKY, et al. Advanced dementia: an integrated homecare programme. BMJ Support Palliat Care 2019;1–10. https://doi.org/10.1136/bmjspcare-2019-001798.

Moving?

Make sure your subscription moves with you!

To notify us of your new address, find your **Clinics Account Number** (located on your mailing label above your name), and contact customer service at:

Email: journalscustomerservice-usa@elsevier.com

800-654-2452 (subscribers in the U.S. & Canada)
314-447-8871 (subscribers outside of the U.S. & Canada)

Fax number: 314-447-8029

Elsevier Health Sciences Division
Subscription Customer Service
3251 Riverport Lane
Maryland Heights, MO 63043

*To ensure uninterrupted delivery of your subscription, please notify us at least 4 weeks in advance of move.

Printed and bound by CPI Group (UK) Ltd, Croydon, CR0 4YY

03/10/2024

01040469-0012